Springer Series on Social Work

Albert R. Roberts, PhD, Series Editor

Advisory Board: Gloria Bon⸺ ⸺kman, PhD, Elaine P. Congress, DSW, Sl⸺ ⸺t J. Greene, PhD, Jesse Harris, DSW, C. A⸺

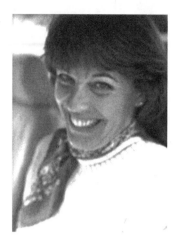

Elise Beaulieu, MSW, ACSW, LICSW, a graduate of Boston College, is currently an Assistant Professor at North Shore Community College. She has served on the faculty at other colleges as well. She is presently the Chair of NASW's Nursing Home Committee and provides consultation social work services to area nursing facilities. She has over 25 years of geriatric and nursing home expeience, including Visiting Nurses, housing, and social services in home care.

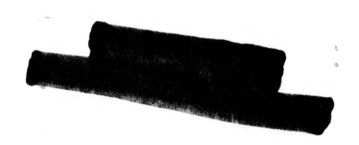

A Guide for Nursing Home Social Workers

Elise M. Beaulieu, MSW, ACSW, LICSW

 Springer Publishing Company

Copyright © 2002 by Springer Publishing Company, Inc.

All rights reserved

No part of this publication may be reproduced, stored in a retrieval system, or transmitted in any form or by any means, electronic, mechanical, photocopying, recording, or otherwise, without the prior permission of Springer Publishing Company, Inc.

Springer Publishing Company, Inc.
536 Broadway
New York, NY 10012-3955

Acquisitions Editor: Emily Epstein
Production Editor: Jeanne Libby
Cover design by Susan Hauley

02 03 04 05 06/5 4 3 2 1

Beaulieu, Elise M.
    A guide for nursing home social workers / Elise M. Beaulieu.
        p. cm. — (Springer series on social work)
    Includes bibliographical references and index.
    ISBN 0-8261-1533
    1. Medical social work—United States   2. Social work with the aged—United States.
3. Nursing homes—United States. I. Title. II. Springer series on social work
(Unnumbered)
HV687.5.U5 B4 2002
362.1'0425—dc21   2001040066
                                                                              CIP

Printed in the United States of America by Maple-Vail Book Manufacturing Group.

This book was made possible through the consistent encouragement and support of my husband, Robert, and my parents, Mary Gene Martini and Herman E. Martini. Special thanks to the NASW Nursing Home Social Work Committee who also supported this work.

Contents

Part IV. Surveys

Part V. Diagnoses and Treatment

Part VI. Legal Representatives for Residents

Part VII. Ethics

Part VIII. Community Liaisons

Part IX. Problems and Solutions

Part X. Standardized Forms

PART ONE

Introduction

CHAPTER ONE

Introduction to Social Work in Nursing Facilities

The role of social work in nursing facilities is a very important one in the lives of residents, families, and staff. Whether the nursing facility is called a nursing home, a long-term care center, or a subacute care or rehabilitation center, the social worker is an essential, vital member of the health care team. As in other settings, social workers in nursing home settings use professional casework skills to help people in particular times of crisis and stress. As a contributing member of the interdisciplinary team, the social worker provides an opportunity for residents and families to examine problems, mobilize existing resources or refer to resources that are more appropriate, and develop positive resolutions.

The first book about nursing home social work was sponsored by the National Institute of Mental Health in 1974: *A Social Work Guide for Long Term Care Facilities*, by Elaine M. Brody and contributors. A wonderful resource for social workers, this work contained an overview of long-term care facilities and explained the functions of the social worker in the facility. Another book written about nursing home social work was *Gerontological Social Work Practice in Long-Term Care*, edited by George S. Getzel and M. Johanna Mellor (1983). This book discussed the practice demands of social workers in nursing homes and home care, acute care, and rehabilitation settings.

The Guide's purpose is to improve the services to residents of nursing homes and their families through improvement of social work knowledge and skills. Changes in the long-term care health system have helped to make the role of the nursing home social worker more important to residents and families in the new millennium. In many facilities, however, the position of the nursing home social worker has been defined by other disciplines or subject to multiple interpretations, thus making the role amorphous and vague.

The Guide's chief objectives are

- to support professional social workers in the interdisciplinary setting and encourage them to provide directly for the mental health and psychosocial needs of the residents and families;

- to help define and clarify the role of the social worker in today's nursing facility;
- to provide specific resources and supplemental material to assist the social worker in his or her job;
- to provide education and increased awareness of the benefits of the social work role in nursing homes for other professionals (administrators, nurses, physicians, etc.) in the field.

MYTHS AND REALITIES ABOUT SOCIAL WORK IN NURSING FACILITIES

There are a number of myths surrounding nursing homes, social work, and the needs of residents and families. The following are some of the myths and the associated realities addressing some of the perceptions about long-term care, the older population, and social work.

1. **Myth:** Long-term care *only* refers to nursing facilities.
Reality: Long-term care today refers to much more than just a nursing facility. It comprises a large continuum of care services provided to individuals in their homes and assisted living settings. Long-term care has developed and expanded over the past 3 decades to include many and even coexisting multiple options for the older person and families. There are a wide range of agencies, both private and public, that offer an array of community resources to match the needs of the elder and the family. For example, Area Agencies on Aging (AAA) are nationally designated sites that act as clearing houses for information and services about aging for local, state, and federal programs.

Levels of care, that in previous cases may have referred only to the differences within a nursing home facility now address a continuum of care, such as home care (nursing, rehabilitative, home health aide, or companion care), adult day care, respite care, congregate housing, continuing care retirement communities, assisted living centers, residential care settings, intermediate care facilities, and skilled nursing facilities (*Long term care report,* 1998, May). Payment for these services range from private payment and insurance supplements to public funds.

Case management services to families and elders, both private and public, can offer foster care settings, hospice care, and an array of in-home services and resources such as Meals on Wheels, money management, guardianship services, extensive or moderate home health care, respite care, protective services, homemaker services, legal aid, and nursing home eligibility evaluations.

2. **Myth:** Nursing home care is inevitable for all elderly.
Reality: Although the United States has over 15,000 nursing homes (SMG Marketing Group Inc., 2000), only about 4.41% of the population over 65 are presently using a nursing home. This figure (4.41%) varies state by state with some states, like Minnesota, having 7.59% of those over 65 in nursing facilities while others, such as Nevada, have 2.03% in nursing homes (AOA, 2001). Statistics from 1997 also indicate that the median length of stay in a nursing home was 63 days (Gabrel, 2000).

Oregon's LTC System: A Case Study, by the National LTC Mentoring Program (Kane, Ladd, Kane, & Nielsen, 1996) discusses the role of the nursing facility as the last part of the continuum of care for the disabled and elderly. This study discusses how the state, through Oregon's Senior and Disabled Services Division (SDSD) developed a plan that supported greater home and alternative services, reducing the use of nursing homes. Today, the Oregon Health Care Association is much more in harmony with the realities of the LTC system. Interviews with representatives of both nursing home associations indicate that the Oregon nursing home industry has decided to become a part of the state's LTC philosophy.

Oregon's nursing home industry decided to become a part of the state's LTC philosophy. Some nursing homes are specializing in subacute care, while others are expanding with assisted living-like environments that emphasize privacy, dignity, choice, and independence. Many nursing homes are becoming much more active in their communities and are developing the role of being a resource to their home and community-based care providers.

A new, proactive philosophy was developed to address the shifting desired outcomes of providing necessary care and services, at the least cost and in the least confining situation. Three of the new concepts are

Shared responsibility—A concept that advocates establishment of mutual expectation between LTC consumers and providers about exercising control over and assuming a degree of responsibility for the results of decision making.

Bounded Choice—A concept that advocates impose limits on the individual's choice of services based on service capacity, societal norms, and available resources.

Managed Risk—A concept that advocates a formal process of negotiating a plan to address an individual's decisions or preferences, to decrease the probability of poor outcomes or of putting others at risk for adverse consequences.

3. **Myth:** Social workers have always had clearly defined roles in nursing facilities.
Reality: Before 1987, the role and position of the social worker in the nursing home was decided by individual states. This created a wide variation of responses from the nursing home industry to the psychosocial needs of the residents. Some states did not mandate a facility to have a social worker as a part of the staff. Other states provided very clear designations of the social worker's role and involvement.

Essentially, social work has changed along with the evolution of nursing homes. Some social workers in nursing homes had very ill-defined roles that varied from facility to facility. One job description, while vague in many of the duties of the social worker, specifically dictated a minimum age: "She (the social worker) must be at least 21 years of age." Social workers, even in the large nursing home settings were frequently part-time workers. Areas of responsibility also differed for social workers even within the same state. Sometimes social workers became responsible for being part-time bookkeepers or activity directors to "justify full-time" positions in facilities.

In 1987 the federal government through OBRA (The Omnibus Reconciliation Act of 1987, P.L.100-203, the Nursing Home Reform Act) under "Quality of Life" created a national umbrella of care for residents in nursing homes. This included a range of mental health and social services for nursing facility residents and a specific mandate for social workers as a part of the facility staff. This mandate addressed the need to have a qualified social worker in a facility of over 120 beds, and the requirements of minimal education and experience necessary for this position, i.e., "A bachelor's degree in social work or a bachelor's degree in a human service field including but not limited to sociology, special education, rehabilitation counseling, and psychology; and one year of supervised social work experience in a health care setting working directly with individuals" (OBRA, 1987).

4.   **Myth:** Social workers in nursing facilities do not need to be highly skilled to provide social services to residents and families.
Reality: Social workers need to be knowledgeable about, and skilled in assessing residents who have multiple needs and multiple diagnoses. For example, the Department of Social and Behavioral Sciences at the University of California San Francisco (1999) indicated that 41.4% of the nation's nursing home residents have reported dementia. This percentage varied from 31.9% in Illinois to 54.6% in Maine. For residents with other psychiatric conditions, other than organic mental syndromes such as schizophrenia, mood disorders, and other problems, the national average is 13.8%. The percentage of conditions varied from 4.1% in Hawaii to 20.5% in Louisiana and Ohio.

> A logical place to begin to enhance mental health and psychosocial services is with trained and educated social workers. There is no other professional whose members are trained to handle the functions required by HCFA's OBRA mandate: to assess and treat mental health needs and to enhance quality of life. The education of professional social workers seeks to prepare them to carry out these functions, including providing psychosocial services and counseling to patients and their families and to afford residents dignity when they are dying. (O'Neill & Rosen, 1998)

5.   **Myth:** Medical care and quality of life are the same.
Reality: Since the introduction of OBRA Regulations in 1987, there has been an increased amount of attention to and recognition of the quality of life for residents in nursing facilities. In the past, institutional settings have not always focused on the individual needs of residents or the unique issues of family members.

The issue of quality of life in nursing facilities is highly important to social services in their role with residents and families. In a fall 1998 panel discussion, Rosalie Kane, DSW, Professor of Public Health at the University of Minnesota, discussed some key issues in quality of life indicators:

> Structure and process indicators, aspect of the physical environment and the facility operations, flexibility in rules and procedures and choices offered to resident are important. Staff communication patterns with residents are

particularly important to consider in assessing a facility's quality of life. A homelike environment on a residential scale is also an important quality of life consideration. In an ideal environment everybody should be offered a private room with a private bath.

6.   **Myth:** Nursing homes have always been large, institutional facilities offering comprehensive care to rehabilitate elders or disabled people.
Reality: In the early 1960s nursing facilities appeared to be different from today's centers. Their size was smaller, averaging less than 120 beds, they commonly had resident rooms with 3–4 beds, there was often little space dedicated to office or management, and recreation areas and rehabilitation rooms were often much smaller, if they existed at all. The emphasis of these early institutional homes was "total institution" with little effort to be homelike.

Today facilities are physically larger than in the past. There are approximately 15,130 nursing homes in the United States. Only 9.8% of these nursing facilities have fewer than 50 beds. Care Scout (2001) indicates the average number of nursing home residents per state varies between West Virginia where there is an average of 169 residents in a facility to Tennessee where there is only an average of 57 per nursing home. Of the current data in 1999, 19.1% of nursing homes had more than 151 beds (SMG Marketing Group, Inc., 2000).

7.   **Myth:** Studies of nursing homes and facility staff have included social work.
Reality: Although there have been many studies about nursing homes, nursing staff, and the care of residents, the role of the social worker has not had much specific attention. Current national and state ombudsman reports include a variety of areas, but blend social services with activities as one heading, making it difficult to determine the impact of the specific role of the social worker.

These struggles have initiated some more current inquiries. In a July 1998 report, John O'Neill and Anita L. Rosen addressed the need for professional social work in the "delivery of mental health and psychosocial services to vulnerable residents of the nation's 17,000 skilled-nursing homes." (p. 5)

Their report further stated,

Some policy and advocacy issues suggested by this project include

- adequate enforcement of OBRA's requirement for quality of life and mental health services;
- clear delineation of scope of practice issues by HCFA in relation to education and credentialling for social services, social work, medical social work, and clinical social work;
- expansion of the availability and access to clinical social work consulting services for nursing home residents and staff; and,
- attention to the substantial mental health needs of SNF residents by policymakers, payors, and regulators.

In Massachusetts, nursing home social workers were polled in 1998, 1999, and 2000, about social worker experience, educational and salary levels, concerns about the job, and long range commitment to the profession. Highlights of the results have indicated stabilization in social worker experience: Fifty-one percent of the social workers reported having over 5 years of experience in the nursing home field. In the year 2000, Massachusetts nursing home social workers were also more likely to have advanced degrees, with 52.70% holding MSWs and 64% earning over $38,000 annually (Beaulieu, 1998, 1999, 2000).

In 1998, 80% of the social workers expressed concerns about ethical issues relating to their role in the facility. The ethical concerns focused upon the practice gaps in the ability to spend adequate individual time with residents and families, run groups, and provide appropriate follow-up care with residents and families. In spite of these practice difficulties, 75% of social workers in the same survey indicated they were satisfied with their profession as a nursing home social worker (Beaulieu, 1998, 1999, 2000).

The ongoing need for social workers in long-term care institutions is very clear. Social workers are needed within all phases of institutional life, from admissions through discharge. It is hoped that this Guide will provide some of the necessary supports and assistance needed by social workers as they pursue their profession of helping residents, families, and others involved in long-term care. Although every effort has been made to provide accurate information and resources, this book simply represents an introduction to the information available at the present time. Social workers should always investigate current rules and regulations regarding their role, and in turn provide the most current information or resources to residents and family members.

REFERENCES

Administration on Aging. (March 2001). *Percentage of elderly in nursing homes.* [On-line]. Available: http://www.aoa.gov/aoa/hcbltc/profiles/65nhpct.html

Beaulieu, E. (1998, 1999, 2000). Massachusetts nursing home social workers survey. Unpublished data.

Brody, E. M. (1974). *A social work guide for long term care facilities.* Rockville, MD: U.S. Department of Health, Education and Welfare. Public Health Service Alcohol, Drug Abuse, and Mental Health Administration. National Institute of Mental Health.

CareScout. (July, 2001). Average number of nursing home resident in a nursing home by state. [On-line]. Available: http://www.carescout-elderanswers.com/resources/nursing home/av no residents.htm

Gabrel, C. (2000). Characteristics of elderly nursing home current residents and discharges: Data from 1997 national nursing home survey. Advance Data. *Vital and Health Statistics,* No. 312.

Getzel, G. S., & Mellor, M. J. (1983). *Gerontological social work practice in long-term care.* New York: Haworth Press, Inc.

———. Nursing facilities, staffing, residents, and facility deficiencies. 1993–1999. Department of Social & Behavioral Sciences. University of California San Francisco. Page 45.

Kane, R. L., Ladd, R. C., Kane, R. A., & Nielsen, W. J. (1996). *Oregon's LTC System: A Case Study by the National LTC Mentoring Program.* University of Minnesota School of Public Health Institute for Health Services.

Kane, R. A. (Fall 1998). *Ask residents about quality: Getting serious about quality of life in nursing homes.* Panel presentation at San Francisco, CA (American Society on Aging).

Long term care report: Care options for elders and their families. (May 1998). *Institute for Long Term Care Policy, 1*(1). [On-line]. Available: http://www.nasw-de.orgNASW/shf.htm

Omnibus Budget Reconciliation Act of 1987, P.L. 100-203, 101 Stat. 1330.483.15.

O'Neill, J., & Rosen, A. L. (1998). *Professional social work services in skilled nursing facilities: Survey of current practice and recommendations.* National Association of Social Workers.

SMG Marketing Group Inc. (2000). *Staffing.* Aventis Managed Care Digest Series. [On-line]. Available: http://www.managedcaredigest.com/is2000/is2000c03s06g01o02.html

CHAPTER TWO

The Changing Face of Nursing Home Social Work

Nursing home social work has continued to change and evolve with the requirements of regulatory agencies, and the public and the internal structure of facilities. National trends of gerontological social work in a National Association of Social Workers (NASW) survey indicate that "39.7 percent of social workers work in health care facilities, 22.5 percent work in social service agencies, 9.1 percent work at colleges or universities, 7.7 percent work in private practice, 5.3 percent work in mental health facilities, and 14.8 percent work in other settings" (Lee, 1999).

The trends noted in the 3 years of surveys of Massachusetts seem to represent the national picture of long-term care nursing facilities in part, and also the trends in the greater Boston area. One of the pictures that emerges in overall changes is in the size of the facility. As with the rest of the country, Massachusetts's facilities are being represented by larger facilities. There are a declining number of facilities overall.

"National estimates indicate that some 16,700 nursing homes had a total of 1.8 million beds and served more than 1.5 million residents during the period July through December 1995. The number of nursing homes decreased 12.6 percent since the 1985 survey while beds in these facilities increased by 9 percent. Data from the National Health Provider Inventory (NHPI) support this decrease in the number of nursing homes and increase in the number of beds over the past few years." (Strahan, 1997, p. 2)

Social work practice in nursing homes has rarely been researched. This study provides insight into social worker's spheres of influence and distinguish between the relative influence of social workers who provide only direct social services and those whose roles include administrative responsibilities. Administrative responsibilities augment the influence of the social work role. Nearly all directors of social services provided direct services. The same may not be true of administrators of nursing and of the facility itself. The social work role is rather narrow and focused; administrative responsibilities broaden the influence and empower the social worker. Social workers have more influence over and less rigidity in their daily lives. Similarly social workers also have more influence on personnel decisions when the administrator has greater decision-making autonomy. Together, these findings suggest that social workers play a crucial role in empowering residents through increasing their autonomy (Kruzich & Powell, 1995).

HOW DOES THE LARGE SIZE OF THE FACILITY AFFECT THE SOCIAL WORKERS?

With larger facilities, there is generally an increase in the number of social workers in the facility. OBRA regulations require a full-time social worker in a facility of 120 beds or larger. In facilities having 140 or more beds, generally there are two social workers providing services.

Facilities are often large and may include subacute units where the fast pace of admissions, treatment, and discharge require a different level of staffing. In addition, some of the larger facilities may also have a separate Alzheimer's unit, also necessitating additional staff levels. There was an almost 10% decline in single-headed social work departments from 1999 (37.86%) to 2000 (27.27%). The two social work department has increased from 39.89% in 1998 to 37.86% in 1999 to 48.95% in 2000 (Beaulieu, 1998, 1999, 2000).

Frequently these new large facilities hiring social workers will look for candidates with an MSW degree. This practice reduces or eliminates the MSW consultant role (required by Massachusetts state law for bachelor level social workers). The consultant has traditionally provided social work expertise as well as educational resources to the nursing facility. The social worker with a consultant avoided professional isolation in the multi-disciplinary setting. (See also Chapter 7, Consultation in the Nursing Home.)

WHAT IMPACT HAVE THESE CHANGES MADE ON SOCIAL WORKER SALARY?

The salary changes have been reflected over the past few years. There was an increase of 10.07% in social workers who earn over $45,760 annually from 1999 to 2000 (Beaulieu, 2000). This result can be attributed to several factors: increasing the level of education and license level for social workers, the "hot" economic situation in Boston area, and the economic adjustment of social workers' salaries coming more into line with other department heads in nursing facilities and OBRA regulations.

It is not clear that social worker salaries have risen equally in other parts of the country. The use of social work designees in many states is reflective of the efforts of the nursing home industry and states to keep overall costs down. The lower salaries do not attract seasoned, professional social workers.

WHAT IS THE STATUS OF THE BSW SOCIAL WORKER IN NURSING HOMES?

OBRA has mandated that nursing facilities employ a full-time social worker with a minimum of a bachelor's degree in social work or a related field, and experience with older people. Since 1999, however, the BSW educated social worker has declined in numbers in the Massachusetts nursing home field by 11.96%! The decline of BSW social workers in this field is puzzling. It may be these social workers are finding employment in other areas, or if they are working with the elderly, it is in the arena of home care, community elder services, or assisted living facilities.

These figures can also be viewed as a result of social workers with MSW degrees out-ranking those with BSW degrees in applying for employment in a nursing home. Although education may well have an impact upon the choice of both the MSW and the BSW in area of training and major, there are few BSWs who have internships in nursing homes Ji Seon Lee (1999, p. 5) notes that "Among BSW programs, only 9% offer concentrations in aging even though the majority of BSWs work with elderly people." This certainly is an area for further study and review.

WHAT HAS HAPPENED ON THE NATIONAL LEVEL TO NURSING HOME SOCIAL WORKERS?

In the national arena, nursing home social work has not fared well in many states. California, Idaho, Arkansas, North Carolina, Kansas, Missouri, Tennessee, and Connecticut all allow social work designees to perform the social work role in nursing homes. In fact, Idaho's recent amendment to the Social Work Act that had delineated social work licensing in the state, created a separate and permanent section for social work designees in the nursing home and health care field (House Bill No. 604, 2000). The use of designees does not conform to the federal statute of OBRA. Nursing homes across the country require licensing and certification for virtually all other professions providing care for residents and families.

HOW DOES EXPERIENCE PERTAIN TO NURSING HOME SOCIAL WORK?

The overall decline in experience in the Massachusetts field has been an interesting observation in these surveys. Social work in nursing facilities is an exceptionally unique occupation requiring extensive knowledge of systems, family, community, and the nursing home industry, as well as expertise in working with aging clients. Some view these social work positions as being less than "clinical," or more mechanical and secretarial. While there is strong evidence in support of the amount of increasing paperwork, social work practice in nursing homes provides much more than a signature. However, for many nursing home social workers, the experience provides the training ground for future work as independent clinicians or for moving into other areas of social work with more prestige.

IS DOCUMENTATION AN ISSUE FOR NURSING HOME SOCIAL WORKERS?

The area of documentation is an ongoing and complex problem of nursing facilities. More and more time seems to be spent on "proving" work. From the

Minimum Data Set (MDS) to Resident Assessment Protocol (RAP), to follow-up notes, histories, and assessments, social workers as well as other staff members are pushing paper at an ever-increasing rate. In the 1998 survey several questions addressed documentation:

- The amount of documentation for social service in the facility is "normal": 58.33% Agreed.
- The documentation is meaningful to the charts: 55.78% Agreed.
- Social service documentation coordinates with other disciplines: 57.57% Agreed.
- Social service documentation can be completed: 60.60% Agreed.

In 2000 the survey attempted to determine how much time was spent in documentation. Just over 72% stated that they spent over 10 hours a week in documentation, and 47.15% spend over 14 hours a week in documentation. Obviously social workers are sacrificing time with residents in order to meet the requirements of documentation, and this is true of all disciplines involved with residents.

HOW DO SOCIAL WORKERS IN NURSING HOMES VIEW THEIR LONG-RANGE COMMITMENT TO THE PROFESSION?

The number of social workers who wish to stay in the profession of nursing home social work for the next 5 years has changed slightly. In 1998, 41.47% of social workers felt positively about remaining in the profession. The 2000 survey revealed that 45.9% of the social workers wanted to remain in their positions for the next 5 years. This indicates a slightly increased level of satisfaction, despite some continued issues and problems.

In summary, these surveys offer the opportunity to study the demographics of the profession of nursing home social work. The surveys also present current trends, particular concerns, and insights into dilemmas faced by nursing home social workers, for example, ethical issues (Beaulieu, 1998, 1999). The information gathered can be utilized in issues of advocacy for practice standards; promoting adequate, fair salaries; and demanding adequate training/consulting. Documentation remains an obvious ongoing issue for the health care professions as a group. It can be an uniting issue for all professionals in the field to advocate for sensible, realistic methods of verifying service provided.

COMMENTS FROM SOCIAL WORKERS FROM THE 2000 SURVEY

Just added up the Direct Service hours above (in the survey) and wow, it's well over 40 hours! Guess I'm not surprised.

Too much documenting! Social workers are becoming a rare commodity in nursing homes. Now is the time for professionals to demand an increase in salaries for social workers!

Too much paperwork, not enough time to spend with residents and families. Need to reevaluate the need for all this paperwork. It is stressful for all staff at nursing facilities, not just social services.

Too many (MSW) social workers settle for too little money. It is the fault of the profession. I would not take a job for less than $45,000 per year.

I may be exaggerating time spent directly with residents and understating time spent with paperwork. I just couldn't bring myself to admit it on paper!

As a post-acute unit social worker, more time seems to be spent with crisis intervention with families, family dynamics, and helping staff than with challenging patients/families.

COMPARISON OF SURVEYS OF NURSING HOME SOCIAL WORKERS: 1998, 1999, 2000

Percentage With Social Work Experience:

	2000	1999	1998
Less than one year	9.92	11	7
1–2 Years	14.18	9	18
3–5 Years	24.82	23	25
5–7 Years	15.60	18	9
8+ Years	35.36	38	40

Percentage With Educational Degrees:

	2000	1999	1998
Bachelor's Degree	24.32	23.57	25.37
BSW	15.54	24	27.5
MSW	52.70	42	38.80
Other	7.44		

Percentage—Length of Time for Present Employment:

	2000	1999	1998
Less than 5 years	76.87	78	79.54

Percentage—Salaries:

	2000	1999
Per Hour and Annual		
$10.00–12.00 ($20,800–24,960)	0	2.1

$12.50–15.00 ($26,000–31,200)	5.59	11.5
$15.50–18.00 ($32,240–37,440)	30	28.05
$18.50–21.00 ($38,480–43,680)	39.16	43.16
$22.00+ ($45,760+)	25.17	15.10

Percentage of Annual Salaries for 1998:

$10,000	4.1
$11,000–20,000	12.3
$21,000–30,000	18.97
$31,000–40,000	46.66
$41,000+	17.94

Percentage—Hours Allocated for Social Service in the Facility in 2000 Survey:

Less than 20	21–32	33–40	41–50	51–80	81–100
13.28	9	19.53	7	31.25	17.96

Percentage Number of Social Workers in the Facility:

	2000	1999	1998
One	27.27	37.86	33.83
Two	48.95	37.86	39.89
Three	14.48	17.86	23.23
Four	6.99	5.7	3

Percentage—License Level:

	2000	1999	1998
LSWA	1 (number)		2 (number)
LSW	38.62	33	50.76
LCSW	34	33	31
LICSW	26.89	20	16.24

Percentage—"Do you want to be a nursing home social worker in 5 years?"

	2000	1998
Yes	45.96	41.57
No	30.64	33.14
Leave SW Profession	23.38	
Not Answered		30.87

REFERENCES

Beaulieu, E. (1998, 1999, 2000). Massachusetts nursing home social work surveys. Unpublished data.

Kruzich, J. M., & Powell, W. E. (1995). Decision-making influence: An empirical study of social workers in nursing homes. *Health & Social Work, 20*(3), 215–223.

House Bill No. 604. (2000). *House Bill No. 604, as amended in the Senate.* [On-line].
    Available: http://www3.state.id.us/oasis/2000/HO604.html
Lee, J. S. (1999). Quick facts on gerontological social work. Section On Aging.
    NSAW, 1(1), 5.
Strahan, G. W. (January 1997). An overview of nursing homes and their current
    residents: Data from the 1995 national nursing home survey. Advance Data. *Vital
    and Health Statistics,* No. 280.

PART TWO

Social Work in Nursing Facilities

CHAPTER THREE

Basic Orientation

HOW IS THE ROLE OF THE SOCIAL WORKER IN THE LONG-TERM CARE FACILITY DEFINED?

The role of the social worker in the long-term care (LTC) setting has been delineated in many ways. Primarily, social work in nursing homes can be defined to include

- psychosocial
- counseling
- resource allocation
- advocacy
- planning and treatment
- mediation

It requires specialized knowledge of

- aging
- medical and mental health diagnoses
- medical diagnoses
- nursing care
- training

In long-term care, the social worker works with the resident and family frequently from pre-admission through the resident's stay to discharge. LTC social workers need to have the astute skills and the ability to provide succinct differential assessments about residents. A view of the resident that is unique to social service is developed through observation, interaction with the resident, significant family members, past medical diagnosis, medical history, and contributions of the team. This helps in meeting the resident's needs while in the placement.

WHAT IS MEANT BY THE PSYCHOSOCIAL NEEDS OF THE LTC RESIDENT?

The psychosocial needs of the resident refer to the psychological and the social aspects of a resident's life. An acute illness or an exacerbation of chronic disease almost always precipitates an admission to the nursing facility setting. The significance of placement therefore encompasses, but is not limited to, the areas of identified physical ailments, change in how care is given and received, the physical relocation of the person and their belongings, as well as how the resident perceives himself and these changes. The social worker captures the essence of these qualities, helping the resident and also the team to expand their understanding of the dynamics involved in the placement.

HOW ARE THE KEY SOCIAL WORK PERSPECTIVES USED?

First and primarily, the identified client in the LTC setting is always the resident. Equally important is the notion that the social worker starts "where the client is," that is, a resident in a nursing facility. In addition, though the resident's family or significant others and their diverse needs may engage the social worker in ancillary tasks, the focus remains on the resident as the client. Residents bring to the LTC a range of issues and problems, some of long standing and others of a more recent nature.

For example, if the resident is admitted for brief treatment and rehabilitation of a fractured hip and shares a history of childhood physical abuse, the social worker may choose to suggest a referral to a community mental-health counseling center for follow-up after the resident's discharge. On the other hand, if the resident's recent loss of a spouse impedes her rehabilitation progress with physical therapy, the social worker may intervene immediately with either direct service or referral to the facility mental-health clinician. In this regard, the social worker in the nursing home setting actually brings professional judgment, the *casework perspective*, to the resident and her problems.

The focus on the

> innate worth of the individual is an extremely important, fundamental characteristic of casework. It is this ingredient that makes it possible to establish the relationship of trust that is so essential for effective social work treatment. From it grow two essential characteristics of the caseworker's attitude toward his client; first *acceptance and second, respect for the client's right to make his own decisions—often referred to as self-determination.* (Hollis, 1972)

Florence Hollis (1972) further discussed the social worker's acceptance of the client or resident with an attitude of warm good will and without criticism for socially inappropriate behavior. She stated the issue of providing the opportunity for the client to make choices within the confines of the presenting reality. For example:

> *A resident, Mr. Cranshaw, 93 years old, who was admitted to the nursing facility from another facility, began to complain about a myriad of tiny details. Some of the issues were remedied quickly, such as a telephone; but others, such as seeing other confused residents, and the color of the paint in the hallway, were components of institutional life. Mr. Cranshaw demanded angrily to return to his previous setting,*

although this was not possible because the bed had already been filled. Outraged at being denied his immediate wishes, the resident yelled at the nursing staff and complained that the social worker was "useless." In an effort to appease him, the facility administrator offered Mr. Cranshaw a private room, but he refused, preferring to remain in his double room and complaining about his roommate. After several weeks of reassurance, consistent kindness, and offers of realistic options for meeting his care needs, Mr. Cranshaw had fewer complaints and decided to remain in the facility.

To be effective for the resident, the social worker in the LTC facility must blend this casework perspective and include multiple areas of the resident's life. In meeting with a resident, the social worker provides an assessment that is a recognized tool for assisting with the needs or problems that are presented within the framework of the resident's past and that is based on available present resources. In addition, positive rapport must be established with the facility staff and administration. This emotional affinity can further the understanding between residents and staff through ultimately increasing the quality of care residents receive. Building links with the community establishes the resources necessary for the care and comfort of nursing home residents.

HOW DO SOCIAL WORKERS ADVOCATE IN NURSING FACILITIES?

The social worker in long-term care provides an important component in the role of advocate for residents. Whether the issue is a room change, transportation issues, or serious financial problems, the social worker's contribution on behalf of the resident is to insure that the resident obtains needed services from the facility or community.

In the facility the social workers can "play a crucial role in empowering residents through increasing their autonomy" (Kruzick & Powell, 1995). By helping the staff to develop attitudes that foster resident independence, individuality, and respect for personal belongings, the social worker diminishes the impact of institutionalization. Advocating resident choice for activities of daily living, such as when to get up in the morning or when to go to bed at night, helps to reduce rigid routines.

Interventions with families are another advocacy role for social workers. Although many families are appropriately effective in their interaction with residents, some families are ineffective, neglectful, and occasionally abusive. It is the social worker's role to assist residents who are having difficulties with their families so that their needs can be met. For example, families frequently retain control of the resident's state allocated personal needs money. At times, this arrangement does not meet the needs of the resident, the family is neglectful in purchasing clothing on a timely basis, or rarely visits. In these circumstances, the social worker's role is to intervene on behalf of the resident. One of the first steps would be to identify to the family the resident's need and the family's expected role. The social worker may present the family with various options and opportunities to meet the obligation and may then choose to take further recourse, with the support of the administration, or legal action if the resident's needs persist because of the negligence of the family.

Social workers in LTC settings frequently bridge the gap between residents and service providers, helping to link people with important resources and opportunities. For example, residents who are being discharged and who are in need of financial assistance for medications may not know about government-sponsored pharmacy programs or may need information about possible adult day health care opportunities and options for transportation in the community. Social workers can also provide links to formal services such as financial advisors and home care agencies.

Advocacy for residents who need help with their medical insurance programs is another area that is a growing need. Health care benefits through Medicare, HMOs, and Medicaid, previously offered and provided as a matter of course, are now being carefully evaluated. If the residents or their families are not assertive, they may not receive their full entitlements. The social worker can help the residents obtain their full benefits by helping to advocate for their needs during their stay and in the discharge setting.

HOW DO SOCIAL WORKERS ENGAGE IN COUNSELING ELDERS IN LTC SETTINGS?

The losses associated with growing older, frailties associated with chronic diseases, and placement in a nursing home can make residents feel sad and vulnerable. Counseling around these issues or others can be provided through (a) the facility social worker; (b) a referral to an outside counseling group contracted by the facility; and (c) the resident's retaining a counselor from outside the facility.

Brief, supportive counseling offers the opportunity for the resident to explore some of the issues that are related to living with others in an institutional setting, having intimate care provided by professional staff, and the loneliness of being separated from their home, familiar routine, family, friends, and community. Counseling can also often include the anticipation of returning to the community and the emotional acceptance of a different level of functioning. Frequently, the nursing facility social worker will provide this type of counseling to residents who are in crisis, who have a short stay, or who are in the subacute section of the facility.

Long-term counseling for nursing facility residents is commonly referred to an outside counseling group. Some social workers refer these cases because they feel they cannot make the extended time commitment necessary to meet with residents for this type of therapy. Other social workers feel that their skills are inadequate for long-term counseling. In addition, nursing home social workers, together with the mental-health team, refer residents to the team for a combination of medication review as well as counseling.

Some residents have an affiliation with a counselor or mental-health service setting that is separate from the facility. Outside mental-health agencies may be retained or sought because of prior treatment issues or because of insurance-based payment. In any case, it is important that the resident have the choice of maintaining this connection and a network of communication needs to be established between the mental-health provider and the facility to address any necessary treatment or needs. The social worker role can be an effective liaison between the two agencies.

WHAT IS CARE PLANNING AND TREATMENT IN THE NURSING FACILITY?

Planning and treatment are important facets of nursing home social work. Throughout the resident's stay in the nursing home, the care plan addresses and provides interventions for problems and needs. It is through the casework skills that social workers in nursing facilities emerge in their discipline of helping residents to become "functional" within the "dysfunction" that brings them to nursing facility admission.

Social workers in long-term care can address a wide range of concrete and emotional issues such as enabling residents to meet their physical and emotional challenges in a positive and constructive manner. The following are some of the areas where the social worker might provide assistance to the resident:

- affiliation
- identity
- invigoration
- privacy
- self-esteem
- space and a place

Entering a new setting can be an anxious situation for many people. To be placed in a nursing facility following an acute physical change and perhaps a hospitalization can create even more of a challenge.

Affiliation, membership, or a sense of belonging is absent immediately for a new resident. How they cope with this change in their lives is based primarily on their flexibility, cognitive status, and the degree to which the environment is "user friendly." The social worker can help by paving the way for the new resident. Simple, friendly introductions to roommates and other residents who are able to communicate with acceptance, introductions to staff, and orientation to the facility give the new resident a sense that this place is kind and helpful.

Privacy can be provided in a multitude of ways. It is important to recognize a resident's need for privacy, both in the physical sense—respecting closed doors or drawn curtains—and the emotional. A resident who does not wish to share certain information with the social worker has the right to withhold that information. As sensitive clinicians, social workers should respect the wishes of the resident who does not want to share private events or feelings. In fact, the social worker can alert others to also respect the wishes of the resident by sharing this choice with the team and indicating an area of sensitivity and the need to provide the requested privacy.

Identity is not as great a problem in the nursing facility as in the hospital, where the patient may be seen simply as "the hip" or "the colonectomy."

However, identity in the sense that the resident had a former life, perhaps significant community standing, or an outstanding work career is often lost in the blur of paperwork, medical diagnoses and, in some cases, because of ageism. The social worker's primary aid in helping to create a well-rounded picture of a resident is the social service history and assessment. The social service history brings to life a resident's past, whether the experience was missionary service in Africa or being a sprint runner on an Olympic team. How does this knowledge shape the way the resident is viewed and treated? Once this information is shared, the staff becomes curious about these past experiences or skills and they will engage the resident in more conversation. This way the social worker can help to bring additional respect for these past accomplishments and help fuse the past with the present.

Self-esteem is exceedingly important to residents. Generally described as the value a person sees in herself, self-esteem can be diminished under multiple stressors. Residents in nursing facilities have had many blows to their independence as well as to their basic body images. Because of illness, disease, and loss they have to make enormous efforts to regain components of their former abilities. In addition, when self-esteem in our culture is measured by our degree of independence, physical handicaps can seriously impede a person's mobility and opportunity to perform everyday tasks with ease. It is the task of the team and, in particular, the social worker to help the resident meet these struggles with positive coping skills.

Invigoration or strengthening the resident's emotional response helps the resident to build upon his abilities. From the social worker's perspective, while the resident is increasing perhaps his ambulating skills, he can also be expanding his emotional skills. The social worker can provide an additional resource to discuss the ups and downs of therapy. Even brief and somewhat casual encouragement and praise for the resident's progress can provide the necessary emotional strength to succeed in his goals.

Space and a place may simply and concretely refer to the need of each resident to have a special place to call her own; the assigned room or bed functions as this formally designated space and place. Labeling doors, beds, dressers, and closets helps orient the resident (and staff, too) to her own possessions. It also designates that this particular space belongs to her as a separate spot in the facility. Most people enjoy having designated space whether it is large or small. For many long-term residents this space is where they can keep their possessions. It is important for the social worker to assist the staff in respecting the possessions of the residents as well as their space. Space and place can also refer to the emotional acceptance and caring of the facility and the staff. Admission to a nursing facility remains a complicated working process. A resident who is made to feel welcome by the staff will feel that her physical needs will be met.

WHAT IS RESOURCE ALLOCATION?

In their work with older residents, social workers help them understand and access their benefit entitlements for such government programs as Medicare A and B, the health plans that provide coinsurance payments and Title XIX (Medicaid), Social Supplemental Income, Social Security Disability Income, as well as HMO or other long-term care insurance benefits. Although the nursing facility social worker does not have to provide full, expert information, it is necessary to have a working knowledge of as many benefit programs as possible to assist with appropriate referrals. This information provides assistance to the resident and family when community discharge is considered, and this information is becoming more critical as older adults are joining HMOs for payment of their stay in the facility.

HOW DOES A NURSING HOME SOCIAL WORKER MEDIATE?

Social workers have a natural role in mediation. Nursing home residents generally enter the facility in the midst of a health crisis. During this period of time, the resident, the family, and even the facility to some extent are in the uncharted waters of a new relationship. Each member of the system—the resident, family, facility staff—has to become acquainted and develop rapport of interaction. At times, these relationships are strained because of miscommunication. The social worker can assist with these issues, helping reduce the problematic communication between residents, families, and staff through routine care-planning meetings and through general advocacy for the resident and regular family meetings.

Settling conflicting issues between family members is not the only area of resident advocacy. Mediation between the resident and outside resources is also important. From health insurance needs to obtaining fair and equitable resources from the community, the social worker can provide assistance.

Mr. Brooker was a 66-year-old, single, childless, legally blind, bilateral above-the-knee amputee who had been a resident of the Sunset Manor Nursing Facility for about 14 months. His Medicaid application was rejected because his friend and power of attorney, Mr. Ives, had misappropriated the money from a savings account and transferred Mr. Brooker's home and property into his own name. After 13 months of nonpayment, the facility's attorneys had sought legal action against Mr. Brooker for nonpayment of his nursing facility bill. Mr. Brooker was very worried and upset about his situation, particularly the potential for discharge. The social worker mediated in this situation on several levels by

- obtaining legal counsel for Mr. Brooker at his expressed wish;
- arranging with the facility to reassure Mr. Brooker that he would not be discharged to the street, as he feared, after receiving the legal notice about his bill;
- discussing the situation with the local Medicaid office and requesting a hearing so that Mr. Brooker's eligibility could be addressed again in the light of this information.

DOES THE NURSING HOME SOCIAL WORKER NEED SPECIALIZED KNOWLEDGE?

Yes. Although a nursing home social worker utilizes accepted social work practice methods, knowledge of the following areas is also important:

- Aging
- Medical and mental-health diagnoses
- Medical procedures
- Nursing care

The field of aging or gerontology is growing by leaps and bounds. It is not the intention of this book to provide the social work practitioner with anything but a sketch of aging. For further information, it is suggested that the social worker purchase current books as resources, regularly attend conferences, and obtain and read journal articles in the areas of interest in aging.

WHAT ADDITIONAL FACTORS DO
SOCIAL WORKERS ADDRESS?

Social work in nursing facilities needs to take into account: the physical, the emotional, and the environmental factors as they are integrated into the older adult's life. As many of the residents of long-term care facilities are but a small sample of the elder population at large, it is important for the social worker to maintain a perspective that the vast majority of older people are living in the community quite independently. It is not "normal" for older people to be in a nursing home. However, it would be remiss to state that all older people are enjoying superb health and are able, without difficulty, to attend to all their day-to-day tasks without support. Many older people suffer from chronic disease ailments, such as osteoarthritis, diabetes, hypertension, and congestive obstructive pulmonary disease (COPD). The dementing disorders are also disease-based and contribute significantly to admission to a nursing facility.

The importance of dignity in the long-term care setting is emphasized by "residents' rights" on the federal government level as well as in the individual states. All residents are entitled to dignity and privacy in their care in nursing homes. The idea of dignity is essential to identifying a person as being someone of worth, or being seen as a person of esteem.

Illness and chronic disabilities and the need for personal care that may or may not be combined with cognitive losses create an enormous impact upon people who are admitted to long-term care settings. Familiar settings and their lives are disrupted dramatically by their acute medical problems and subsequently their reactions may range from withdrawal to the bizarre. The following case illustrates such a situation:

> One newly admitted resident, Mrs. Pike, was very resistant to nursing care. She had multiple diagnoses, including paranoid schizophrenia. She had a large decubitus ulcer on her leg and she insisted that only dressings made of loose cotton batting be used. The social worker worked with the resident and the staff to develop a feeling of trust. Gradually, the resident increased her trust of the staff and she accepted and allowed more appropriate dressings and treatment for her leg ulcers.

It is important that the social worker in the facility be aware of the critical need for dignified treatment. Dignity is important at any age, but this is more significant when there have been so many assaults on the person's independence and sense of worth. Confusion can at times lead a person to think that the resident has reverted to childhood. However, for the confused person, the loss of so many aspects of their lives creates an even greater need to be treated with adult respect and to maintain the remaining self-esteem.

Some key buzzwords to incorporate when working with residents are privacy, respectfulness, choices, confidentiality, adultness, value, and empathy, not sympathy. The social worker can take the lead in assisting staff to think of all residents as grown-ups with the need for choice, respect, and courtesy.

The following are examples of how simple verbal labels can have an impact in the reduction of dignity:

- In one facility a staff member would often refer to residents as a "cutie patootie."
- Another staff member would refer to the residents on her unit as her "kids."
- Some facility staff talk to residents in a special voice, generally of higher pitch, and use language perhaps more suitable for young children and babies.
- "Honey," "sweetie," or "dear" is often used instead of the resident's name.
- Telling a resident to be a "good girl" or "good boy" is inappropriate.

The presentation of confused mental status can perpetuate the myth that the resident has reverted to childhood. The social worker can provide staff education that the residents are not merely "big babies." While the coping strategies in demented residents may be primitive, there remain adult structures. By role modeling and explaining behaviors to residents, social workers can help the staff acknowledge deficits while supporting residents' remaining skills and abilities.

We want to demonstrate our affection and caring for residents in a professional manner. To diminish their adultness encourages childlike behavior and sets an example to other residents that they should ally themselves at the staff level or be subjected to infantilizing. If you have doubts about how we should address residents, think of how you might address the president of your company or the president of your college.

WHAT KINDS OF DIAGNOSES/MEDICAL INFORMATION DOES A SOCIAL WORKER IN LTC NEED TO KNOW?

Although social workers are not directly treating medical conditions in the nursing facility, the knowledge, awareness of the medical conditions that they encounter, and the treatment modalities will be of invaluable assistance to them as well as to residents and their family members.

The elderly resident in the nursing facility is often likely to suffer from both acute and chronic medical conditions. Even though the majority of elders never enter a nursing home, most will suffer from some chronic disease before death. Acute illness or injury is often the reason that a person is hospitalized and a combination of two or more disorders becomes the cluster necessary for placement.

Social workers should be familiar with the more common methods of medical treatment for illnesses and the impact illness has upon the independence of a person. The rehabilitative process (occupational therapy, physical therapy, or speech therapy) is frequently of shorter duration in today's medical system. The social worker should be familiar with the rehabilitation process of the facility and any additional resources for residents.

WHAT IS A CHRONIC ILLNESS?

A chronic illness is a disorder where the symptoms may range from mild or moderate discomfort to severe and debilitating pain or impairment of functioning. Chronic illnesses do not directly lead to a person's death. Often the treatment for a chronic illness is to remediate the symptoms without changing the course of the illness. Some of these diseases are

- arthritis
- heart disease
- diabetes
- hypertension
- chronic obstructive pulmonary disease
- visual impairments, cataracts, glaucoma
- hearing impairment
- sinusitis
- orthopedic impairments
- tinnitus
- renal insufficiencies

WHAT IS AN ACUTE ILLNESS?

An acute illness is generally a disease or disorder that requires fairly quick, direct medical intervention where the person's life could be at serious risk. Disorders might include

- cardiovascular accident or "stroke"
- cancer
- fractures

HOW DOES KNOWLEDGE OF THIS INFORMATION HELP THE SOCIAL WORKER?

The social worker in the nursing facility should be familiar with these disorders, both as the resident receives inpatient treatment as well as during discharge planning. Discharge planning, in particular, requires the social worker to have good working knowledge and information about medical conditions and community supports.

Nursing facility social workers can increase their knowledge by networking with community health providers, attending conferences, reading current literature, and having key resource books available in the facility. In addition, social workers should routinely ask the facility staff about unfamiliar treatments provided for the resident and get their input on how difficult or easy it is for the resident to perform tasks. The following example shows how this kind of knowledge can be applied.

A nursing facility resident who is anticipating returning to the community has a severe visual impairment. He found it impossible to read a self-monitoring glucose device four times a day (frequently a standard protocol for treatment of diabetes). The resident lived in an assisted living setting and this presented a major health care problem because the staff were not "legally" able to help with this medical care need. The situation required a very different discharge strategy by the social worker and by the attending physician. In this case, the physician determined that blood-glucose monitoring would take place through monthly blood samples by a laboratory that made house visits. The resident would continue to take his insulin as prescribed without daily glucose readings. The social worker addressed the revised discharge plan with the resident and the family as well as with the assisted living nurse.

HOW DOES THE SOCIAL WORKER BECOME INVOLVED IN TRAINING?

The social worker in most facilities is the key person for helping the staff recognize and respond to the psychosocial factors associated with placing a person in the nursing facility. He or she has the specialized knowledge of the emotional components of loss, grieving, and adjustment. In addition, the social worker should be familiar with and advocate for residents' rights.

Social workers are frequently asked to present residents' rights to facility staff as a requirement of certified nursing assistants' training and review. Social workers are also routinely asked to provide in-services on other topics that range from advanced directives to abuse, neglect, and mistreatment, ethics, and depression.

As the representative of the nursing facility, the social worker may also be asked to speak to resident family groups, such as family council or even the residents' council about a specific topic pertaining to residents and their placement in the facility. Additional community agencies may ask the social worker to speak to their group, such as the Visiting Nurses, or senior citizens' groups regarding nursing home placement.

Whenever possible, social workers should assist in the internship programs offered by schools of social work. This is a unique opportunity for the student to be mentored into a dynamic, challenging social work career. It also affords the social worker the opportunity to engage in the academic process of combining both theory and practice.

WHAT IF THE SOCIAL WORKER IS UNCOMFORTABLE WITH PUBLIC SPEAKING?

Often social workers are more comfortable in one-on-one settings than in groups. Creativity for training programs is probably more important that being able to stand in front of a group of people and give a lecture. Social workers can help themselves and the process by utilizing case examples or by asking members of the staff to provide examples from their own experience of how they support resident rights. Most staff members are very proud of their work with residents.

If the social worker is fortunate enough to have a consultant, the consultant can substitute for the social worker in a training seminar for the staff. If there is a consulting group, they frequently give in-services or training on specific issues, such as problem-behavior management and depression in older adults, among other things. The group-shy social worker can draw from these resources to provide the staff with the necessary training.

It is also helpful to have resources for the simple reason that in-services frequently require preparation. As social workers are often overwhelmed by their current duties, speaking resources can assist those who are pressured for time.

REFERENCES

Bailey, D. J., & DePoy, E. (1995). Older people's responses to education about advance directives. *Health and Social Work, 20,* 223–229.

Barber, C., & Iwai, M. (1996). Role conflict and role ambiguity as predictors of burnout among staff caring for elderly dementia patients. *Journal of Gerontological Social Work, 26,* 101–117.

Brody, E. (1974). *A social work guide for long term care facilities.* Rockville, MD: National Institute of Mental Health.

Brown, A. S. (1996). *The social processes of aging and old age.* Upper Saddle River, NJ: Prentice-Hall.

Cappeliez, P. (1989). Social desirability response set and self-report depression inventories in the elderly. *Clinical Gerontologist, 9,* 45–52.

Cockerham, W. C. (1991). *This aging society.* Upper Saddle River, NJ: Prentice-Hall.

Davitt, J. K., & Kaye, L. W. (1996). Supporting patient autonomy: Decision making in home health care. *Social Work, 41,* 41–50.

Eliopoulous, C. (1990). *Caring for the elderly in diverse care settings.* Philadelphia: J. B. Lippincott.

Greene, G. J., Jenson, C., & Harper Jones, D. (1996). A constructivist perspective on clinical social work practice with ethnically diverse clients. *Social Work, 41,* 172–180.

Gruzalski, B., & Nelson, C. (1982). *Value conflicts in health care delivery.* Cambridge, MA: Ballinger.

Humphry, D. (1991). *Final exit.* Eugene, OR: The Hemlock Society.

Hollis, F. (1972). *Casework: A psychosocial therapy.* New York: Random House.

Kruzich, J. M., & Powell, W. E. (1995). Decision making influence: An empirical study of social workers in nursing homes. *Health and Social Work, 30*(3), 215–223.

Kubler-Ross, E. (1975). *Death: The final stage of growth.* New York: Simon & Schuster.

Lichtenberg, P. A., & Barth, J. T. (1989). The dynamic process of caregiving in elderly spouses: A look at longitudinal case reports. *Clinical Gerontologist, 9,* 31–44.

Mercer, S. O. (1996). Navajo elderly people in a reservation nursing home: Admission predictors and culture care practices. *Social Work, 41,* 181–189.

Mitchell, C. G. (1998). Perceptions of empathy and client satisfaction with managed behavioral health care. *Social Work, 43,* 404–411.

Potts, M. K. (1997). Social support and depression among older adults living alone: The importance of friends within and outside of a retirement community. *Social Work, 42,* 348–362.

Sheikh, J. I., & Yesavage, J. A. (1986). Geriatric Depression Scale (GDS): Recent evidence and development of a shorter version. In T. L. Brink (Ed.), *Clinical gerontologist.* New York: Hawthorn Press, 165–173.

Witkin, S. (1999). Taking humor seriously. *Social Work, 44,* 101–104.

Woodruff, D., & Birren, J. E. (1975). *Aging.* New York: Van Nostrand.

CHAPTER FOUR

The New Social Worker

Gennifer W. began her job at the 140 bed First Ocean View Nursing Home as Director of Social Services. An organized, experienced geriatric social worker who had worked in a Family Service Counseling Center, Gennifer was surprised to find herself over-whelmed by the myriad of details that were presented in her new job at the nursing facility. Meeting the residents of the facility and discovering their strengths and needs was one component that she enjoyed immensely. However, the range and scope of resident and family issues, the paperwork and the "decision tree" for the state, the OBRA LTC compliance, the staff queries, and the seeming general chaos of minutia of the day-to-day operations of the facility, left her head spinning. Panicked by her observations, Gennifer was fearful she would fail in her new job. Instead of giving up, she began to consider the situation, decided that it might help to think proactively. She started to organize her work time and prioritize the needs of the residents and the facility, thus giving some measure of control to her day.

What *is* the new social worker to do? What responsibility is first, second, third, fourth, etc.? Who can help make those decisions? What will happen if these details are not done on a timely basis because someone "forgot"? (Other members of the staff talked fearfully of state surveys and, in the past, "heads had rolled" when surveys were poor.) How can there be enough time in the day for the social worker to attend to all these situations and the needs of the residents or families, and, of course, document all that has taken place?

It would not be unusual to think that the social worker balancing all these details might be well equipped to have the expertise of a circus juggler, the patience of the Biblical Job, and the concentration and skill of a metropolitan air traffic controller. Our social worker in the vignette was correct in her approach: Proactive organization is vital to getting to know residents and staff and sorting through the details of the ongoing paperwork. Creating lists, developing tracking systems and carving out special time for resident visits, family meetings, documentation, and telephone calls is helpful in addressing the multiple components of documentation. Though the layers of details in the position appear overwhelming, there is pattern, logic, and a general system that can be utilized to help social workers "plow though" and provide good social work to residents and families, and participate with the team.

The decision tree approach is one way to view social work in the nursing home. If Mrs. W., a 78-year-old widow who has a diagnosis of cerebral vascular accident (CVA) with right hemiplegia, and a history of depression that spanned 2 decades with one inpatient psychiatric hospitalization, is admitted to our facility, our initial social service admission assessment and plan will entail a very different response than for Mr. J., 72, married, who is admitted following a right knee replacement, with no previous mental health history. Let's take a look at the decision tree with these two examples:

Mrs. W.
Age: 78
Marital Status: Widowed
Children: 2 sons and 1 daughter
Admitted From: Stoney Memorial Hospital; Days of stay 2/7–2/23
Diagnoses:
   s/p CVA with right hemiplegia
   Ambulating with a cane
   HTN
   Small "healing" ulcer on her right heel
   "Pleasantly Confused" ? of Alzheimer's Disease
   Legal blindness
   Depression (more than 20 years)
   Hospitalized: 1980 at Quilty Psychiatric Facility; Dates are unknown; ? of ECT.
Mental Health:
   Pre-admission OBRA Pre-admission Screening and Annual Resident Review (PAS-SAR) indicates the need for mental health evaluation. Present status at admission: incomplete.
Medicare:
   Eligible with Mass Health back up. LTC Screening Form requested at hospital, sent to LTC office. Telephone approval for 30 days according to admissions coordinator.
Family:
   One son and one daughter of the resident's family live in Colorado. Her eldest son is reputed to be in jail for life in Massachusetts. She has one friend in her Senior Housing apartment complex.
Advance Directives:
   Health care proxy with son in Colorado and a Do Not Resuscitate (DNR) status in hospital, none current.
   The referral from the hospital discharge planner indicates both family and resident anticipate her returning to her apartment with services after recovery.

Where does the social worker begin with this case? What questions need to be answered? What details are needed and what parts, should they become known, should be held in confidence?

One of the first important areas of investigation would be for the social worker to meet Mrs. W. Her presenting picture, on paper, may suggest greater or lesser pathology. The social worker would need to follow up in these areas:

1. Does she understand the admission to the facility?

- The social worker needs to develop a fairly quick rapport with the resident in order to assess Mrs. W.'s cognitive capacity. After establishing this relationship, the social worker will determine her level of understanding of the admission.
- If yes, does she understand her rights and responsibilities as a resident? Has she signed her own admission papers? (Legal issues can develop at this point for competency.)
- If no, what resources are available to her? Has her son or daughter in Colorado been contacted and who will be taking a bigger role? Is there a Durable Power of Attorney? What about a temporary legal guardian for her? How and within what time constraints will the social worker facilitate all this?

2.   Social worker also needs to follow up on the following:

- OBRA PASARR assessment
- Long-term screening from Mass Health
- Resources available for her to return to her home

3.   Mrs. W.'s very brief history from the hospital indicates a son in Massachusetts who has apparently committed a crime for which he is serving a life prison sentence. How relevant will this be in the social service worker's history? (He had been convicted of an organized crime slaying almost 28 years ago and Mrs. W. had visited him once a month up until 2 months ago.) How much history, assuming that this will be a brief admission, does the social worker want to obtain? If Mrs. W stays in the facility longer, how much more history might be needed? Should the social worker think about an addendum to the social service history?

4.   The hospital discharge summary to the long-term care facility indicated that everyone wanted Mrs. W. to return to her apartment. What kinds of services will she need? What agency or agencies can provide this? What choices does Mrs W. need to be aware of? What will the team want to create for a goal in her desire to return to the community?

5.   What about her clothing, shoes, and personal items? Who might the social worker contact about obtaining these? Does the social worker contact the friend in the community without getting permission from Mrs. W.?

6.   How does the social worker complete her MDS sections? Mrs. W. with her observed "confusion" in the acute care setting, appears to be forgetful about her habits in the community. Does the social worker, with permission of the resident, call the local friend? How might the family help? What if the friend is also elderly and disabled?

7.   The plan of care and the RAPS from the MDS will need to be addressed. How will the social worker word her plan of care? What key elements need to be addressed with regard to her stroke; her mental health diagnosis? Does the pre-admission OBRA PASARR screening evaluation fit into a plan of care? How do the social worker and the team address discharge? Who is invited to the admission care plan meeting? What about later meetings and evaluations of the team?

Mr. J
Age: 72
Marital Status: Married
Admitted From: Stoney Memorial Hospital; Days of stay 2/15–2/24
Diagnoses:
   Right total knee replacement
   HTN
   Anxiety
Mental Health:
   Pre-admission OBRA PASARR screening indicates no need for mental health evaluation.
Medicare:
   No, HMO with case management 7-day limited stay.
Family:
   Wife. 70 years old, legally blind, unable to drive.
   Son and daughter-in-law: next-door neighbors to resident.
Advanced Directives:
   None

What questions might the social worker ask in this case? What parts are important to the resident's stay and discharge?

Meeting the resident quickly might be important in this case. Why? Who else in this case will be of importance? How does the social worker help the team meet their goals with the information he or she gleans from the meeting with the resident?

1.   Should the social worker expect the resident to have understood the admission and signed the admission paperwork?

- If yes, does the social worker review the resident's rights and responsibilities again?
- If no (the resident has not signed the admitting papers), does the social worker interpret this? How might this be interpreted? If someone else has signed the admitting paperwork does the social worker review the resident's rights with the resident? Does the social worker discuss advance directives? Why or why not?

2.   The admission is obviously very brief. Does the social worker collect a social service history? Why or why not?

3.   The social worker will need to follow up on

- Available resources from the HMO to return home
- Available community resources for the couple
- Available family resources for both husband and wife

4.   Mr. J.'s admitting diagnoses include "Anxiety." What, if anything, does the social worker address here? Is it necessary for the social worker to review this diagnosis for a "short" admission? When would it be important? When would it not be important?

5.   What, if anything, can be expected from the resident's wife? Does the social worker call her for clothing and necessary items for the resident? How might this be handled?

6.   What would be important to document in this case? What might not be important? Does the social worker create a plan of care?

7.   In documenting in Mr. J's chart, what will the social service focus upon? How will the MDS be completed?

Both these typical long-term care case examples have wide variations in their presentation. At the same time, there are several common threads: focus on the needs of the resident, involvement of family, and a community discharge plan anticipated by the referring hospital. The social worker frequently determines the answers to the case questions through an ongoing problem-solving approach. The unique responses to questions help the social worker formulate the individual resident assessment goals and plan.

The team members, as well as the social worker, must be flexible with their predetermined plan of care for residents. As the treatment process moved forward for Mr. J., it appeared that his discharge date needed to be adjusted to meet his psychological needs and anxiety. Mr. J.'s heightened anxiety and reduced participation in therapy led to a revised discharge date, a week later. On the other hand, Mrs. W. appeared to do remarkably well in the setting. Her previously noted confusion had cleared and she was able to return to her apartment with services 18 days from the date of admission.

Charts and Documentation

WHAT IS THE RESIDENT CHART?

The resident chart is generally a large loose-leaf binder designated with the resident's name and room number on the spine. Inside the chart there are plastic divisions noting each discipline that is involved with the resident in the facility. The chart is a reference for everyone caring for the residents and, in particular, provides the social worker with a source of information about the current disciplines that are involved in the care of the residents as well as the resident's progress toward his goals.

IS ALL THE INFORMATION ABOUT THE RESIDENT IN THE CHART?

No. Some facilities have ancillary binders, to reduce the size of the individual charts. These can contain anything from physician's orders, to care plans, to permission sheets, to psychotherapist's notes. It is important to be aware of where all this information is kept and remember to review it for information pertaining to the resident. There is also generally an "overflow" file that can be kept either at the nurse's station in a drawer or in medical records. This information is generally old or outdated chart data. Occasionally, information can be thinned from the charts improperly and placed there. Also, if a resident has had more than one admission to the facility the previous charts will be in the medical records file for discharged residents.

HOW IS THE CHART GENERALLY ORGANIZED?

A cover sheet or "face sheet," in the first page of the chart tells the reader basic information, such as full name; date of birth; community address; phone number; previous acute care setting if applicable; admitting date; diagnoses; next of kin with names, addresses, and telephone numbers; attending physician(s); admitting payment sources; funeral home preference, if any; all current health insurance numbers; and previous admissions. Following this initial section, the chart can be arranged in sections labeled Admissions, Legal, Physician's Orders, Nursing, MDS, Care Plan, Physical Therapy, Occupational Therapy, Dietary, Consults, Psychiatric Services, Social Service, Activities, and Misc. The information within these sections can be arranged from latest dated and most current in front, to the reverse, the current notes being the last pages in the section. It is important for the social worker to be familiar with the particular setup of information in the chart so as not to make mistakes or improper inferences from dated material.

DOES THE REFERRING FACILITY
PROVIDE ANY INFORMATION?

Yes. If a resident has been transferred from another agency, facility, or hospital, the chart will probably contain *discharge summary* that may include multiple pages from the previous hospital or LTC facility. This information is provided by the sending facility to the receiving facility in order for the resident to receive continuity of care.

There are not any standard requirements about the content for discharge summaries. Some facilities send copies of all testing, hospital evaluations, screenings, and treatment, and a typewritten summary as well; others are much briefer, primarily checklists. As staffing changes occur in the health care industry, referrals have increasingly omitted a social service section.

Attending physicians from the sending or referring facility always need to sign the discharge summary in order for the transfer to be complete. There will usually be a brief dictated note indicating the type of treatment the resident was receiving. As with other referrals, the information contained therein may be very brief or more descriptive.

The nursing facility social worker should review all the information in the discharge summary. It should be reviewed for content, accuracy, and recommendations to the receiving facility. Referrals containing recommendations should be acknowledged in the social worker's admission note. If the recommendations do not seem to fit the situation presented by the resident and the family, this should be addressed. For example, a referral was received with the anticipation that the resident would be discharged to her home following rehabilitation. After the resident completed her therapy, her condition was still not stable for a community discharge and she remained in the facility as a long-term resident. The social worker addressed this change of plans in his notes.

Many disciplines offer a wide range of information about the resident and the rehabilitative process that is important for the social worker to review. For example, the occupational therapist may include a summary that describes the resident's family more clearly, or discusses issues around safety in the home. These components are helpful in the discharge process.

DO OTHER LONG-TERM CARE FACILITIES PROVIDE INFORMATION?

Yes. When there is a transfer from one facility to another, long-term care facilities frequently provide synopses of the resident's stay in the facility. The social worker is obligated to read this material carefully and address, in the social service section of the chart, any and all issues that pertain to the resident's needs. Key areas of importance are emotional and psychosocial issues, or future discharge arrangements. The mood or psychosocial problems of the resident do not necessarily merely appear in the social service section of the referral. Frequently, other disciplines will note problems as well, such as Nursing, Physical Therapy, Dietary, Occupational Therapy, and Speech Therapy.

DOES THE DISCHARGE SUMMARY CONTAIN INFORMATION ABOUT OTHER PREVIOUS HOSPITAL STAYS?

Every facility, whether hospital, subacute, or long-term care, is obligated to provide the receiving facility with all the pertinent information about the resident at the time of discharge to ensure that appropriate care will be continued. Psychiatric/psychological information will be supplied with medical information, though summaries of care and needs, as opposed to copies of notes, will be included. Additional specific information from the sending facility may be requested, with the written permission of the resident or legal representative. Other facilities (hospitals, etc.) that the resident may have stayed in prior to the most recent admission are not allowed to provide information. In fact, a separate signed request for each preceding stay, for each facility, must be made. This ensures resident confidentiality.

WHAT KINDS OF LEGAL DOCUMENTATION CAN BE FOUND IN THE CHART?

Charts can contain a variety of legal information about the resident. Admissions agreements are generally included in the chart as well as the residents agreement to have treatment and care in the facility. Agreements for requests of previous medical information are also held in the chart and may be located in this section. The legal section of the chart can hold documents such as living wills, health care proxies, durable powers of attorney, and guardianship designation. Social workers should be aware of the importance validity of the names and dates on the documents. For example, permission for previous medical information can be only to a specific hospital or for a specific period of time, guardianships can be temporary and expire in 90-days of the date issue, health care proxy designees can be deceased, or no longer interested in the resident (see Chapter 6, Legal Auspices of Social Work).

The specific legal documentation can vary from state to state. It is important for the facility to have copies and to be informed of any and all legal representation of the resident. The social worker should, with the team, review the material on a regular basis, to maintain the current intent. Some legal representation is time sensitive (there is an expiration date). If legal representation has expired, the social worker may need to provide resources for the resident.

WHAT SECTION OF THE CHART DISCUSSES THE MEDICAL TREATMENT?

Charts most often include current physician's orders, current diagnoses, medicines, and orders for specific treatment. It is necessary for the social worker to recognize that physician orders are the primary key to the care of the resident's stay in the facility. It is through the physician's orders the resident receives current medical permission to stay in the facility. Without physician orders, the resident cannot stay in the facility nor be treated by the staff. Orders from the physician include, but are certainly not limited to, such areas as medication, permission to go on activities outings, treatment of physical therapist or occupational therapist, special wound treatments, and psychotherapy, or being seen by a psychiatrist. Changes in orders are generally found in the same section.

In addition, nursing notes describe and address the medical treatment of the resident. Although ongoing specific treatment notes may be in a separate book, the chart will also indicate when a treatment has been performed. If a resident, for example, has a decubitus ulcer, the nursing notes will indicate treatment for this condition. In addition, there are often photos of the condition to indicate the initial stage and the progress through treatment.

Nursing notes also describe from their perspective, the behavior of a resident interacting with caregivers, notes of visitors, resident conflicts, general medical condition, and response to changes in medication or treatment. The writing skill of the nurse, the opportunity to observe and/or document during a particular shift may result in variations of nursing notes for quantity and quality. When possible, social workers should follow-up with the nurse who wrote a note describing a problem with a resident. This enables the social worker to clarify the issues presented.

WHAT OTHER AREAS OF THE CHART ARE IMPORTANT TO THE SOCIAL WORKER?

Other areas of the chart, which are important to the social worker include Consults, Psychiatrist and Psychologists Reports, and the Recreational Therapist. These sections will provide the social worker with the resident's progress toward the specific discipline goals.

The chart will frequently contain the current nursing notes and weekly summaries, as well. The nursing section varies from facility to facility, but primarily nursing notes chart the very specific progress of the resident and both subjectively and objectively report day-to-day happenings in the resident's life.

Nursing notes can be found for all three shifts in the chart, though the amount of reporting may vary from one or two lines to paragraphs. In addition to charts, there are also 24-hour report books that describe residents' issues from one shift to another. As nursing staff observes the resident for a 24-hour period of time, changes in behavior, attitude, and emotional state can be documented from their perspective. The social worker can use these observations to compare his or her own experiences and views of the resident. For example, a resident may be very resistant around personal care performed by the nursing staff, but very conversational and pleasant in "social situations" with professionals, such as the social worker.

HOW DOES THE CHART REFLECT THE BEHAVIORAL ISSUES OF A RESIDENT?

Residents who have special behavioral or psychological issues may also have logs in the chart where the staff notes a resident's behavior during each particular shift. These can be important in filling out components of the MDS. Nursing notes do not necessarily reflect the behaviors noted in the behavioral log. Some charts contain the resident plan of care, the initial admitting MDS, current MDS, RAPs, OBRA, and PASARR screenings as well. (Please see Part II, which discuss these components.) *In some facilities the current copy of this information is in a separate binder.*

WHAT IS CONTAINED IN THE SOCIAL SERVICE SECTION OF THE CHART?

The social work section of the chart should contain an individual social service history and assessment as well as the ongoing notes, which represent the resident's progress toward the outlined established social service goal(s). A complete, thorough social service history and assessment are critical to establishing good care-planning goals and outcomes of the facility stay. Social workers utilize this resident information obtained in a social service history and assessment to complete their sections of the MDS as well.

WHAT IS THE CONTENT OF SOCIAL SERVICE DOCUMENTATION?

The content of notes in the social service section of the chart can vary from facility to facility. Documentation in clinical records serves the purpose of conveying and recording information about residents necessary and helpful for their care and treatment. Charts may, or may not contain highly sensitive information about the resident. All chart records are confidential and should utilize the least amount of sensitive information necessary to convey to the rest of the team the nature and type of issues presenting, as well as the best way to approach the resident.

HOW IS NECESSARY, BUT SENSITIVE, SOCIAL SERVICE INFORMATION CONVEYED IN THE CHARTS?

As with all social work, material presented in the chart by the social worker should demonstrate good professional judgment and adherence to social work ethics. Family issues, staff issues, and resident-to-resident issues need to be documented in a manner that

1. respects and preserves the rights of all involved;
2. conveys objectively the issues relating directly to the resident; and
3. provides a plan of care that is consistent with known, good practice standards.

It is common knowledge that the documenter *never* names another resident in the chart. A note involving two residents might read as follows:

> 5/9   Ethel Jonas and her roommate had a loud verbal disagreement today over an open window in the room they share. Mrs. Jonas complained that she needed fresh air. Her roommate stated that she was cold and wanted the window shut. The social worker met with both residents . . .

It should *not* read:

> 5/9   Ethel Jonas and Janice Brown had a loud, name-calling, screaming fight today over the open window. Janice called Ethel some vulgar names. The social worker met with both residents . . .

While there is a social service note in both charts, neither resident should be named in the other's chart. The first note is a synthesis of the incident; the second note is verbatim reporting. Facility incident reports are also kept in a separate binder, but are not referred to in the resident chart.

Issues presenting around families must be also handled and documented with diplomacy and care, particularly with regard to specific behaviors or knowledge of a family member's actions outside the setting. For example, a social worker who has knowledge about a resident's family member being treated for a mental disorder, would not document this information in the resident's clinical record.

Chart notes should not be used to take out annoyances or frustrations with other disciplines or administration. A simple statement of the fact(s) and the social worker's plan of intervention on behalf of the resident is the important and appropriate content.

WHO CAN READ THE CHART?

Who can read the resident's chart? In general, everyone who is employed by the facility who has a component of care to provide the resident may read the chart. This includes all nursing staff, consults, physicians, nurse practitioners, etc. According to each facility policy, the resident or resident designated family member may read significant portions or the entire chart and obtain copies of the entire chart or particular pieces. The facility ombudsman may also read the chart with the resident's permission. (See also Chapter 29, Confidentiality.)

WHAT ARE THE KEY ELEMENTS IN ANY NOTE?

The social worker should always keep in mind that charts convey information. The following are useful standards in any social work documentation:

- the date of the activity;
- the identifying information about the resident, such as name, age, etc.;
- the purpose of the activity (e.g., reason for the interview, intervention) and a short statement of the major problem identified by the resident and clarified by the worker;
- important facts surrounding the problem;
- how the problem was handled, the service plan, why it was handled that way, and the outcomes;
- what follow-up activities, if any are being planned; and
- comments and questions to discuss with supervisor or another worker.

WHAT ARE THE IMPORTANT PARTS OR COMPONENTS OF THE CHART FOR THE SOCIAL WORKER DOCUMENTATION?

There are major pieces of documentation for the chart for which social workers are responsible: Remember the social worker is a part of the team. The chart serves as information to all team members and should be as accurate and complete as possible.

Pre-admission/admission note—Due within 24–48 hours of admission.

Social service history—The specific due date for a social service history may vary from state to state. Some states have guidelines that state a history is due within 14 days of admission. Other states' guidelines may insist the history be due within the guidelines of the MDS.

Generally social service is also responsible for:

Social service—Plan of care matches the MDS/RAPS, as early as 5–7 days of admission or as late as 14 days from admission.

Discharge plan—Due date matches the care plan.

Quarterly note—Every 90 days, or matching the goals set within the care plan.

Sections of the MDS—Due as set by type of admission. PPS dictates the Medicare schedule. Beyond the Medicare schedule, the MDS is due quarterly and annually, or when there is a resident condition that is recognized as a significant change.

RAPS—Addressing triggered by the MDS sections.

Care plans—Reflecting social service interventions.

WHAT IS A S.O.A.P. NOTE?

SOAP notes are an organizational method of writing about the contact with the resident. The follow is a description of the meaning of SOAP:

S = Subjective content. Often the "S" part of the note, presented in this fashion will begin with a statement or quote from the resident such as: "I have had such a hard day today." The statement is meant to convey emotions that qualify the interaction.

O = Objective content. The "O" component of the note is an objective description of the resident as the interviewer. An "O" might appear as: "The resident was sitting in a chair by the window with her head down. She looked sad, and it appeared that she had been crying, as she was holding a handkerchief and her eyes were red and watery. The chart (nursing note of 3/12) indicated that her pet cat at home had died."

A = Assessment content. The "A" represents the component where the professional makes a summary determination of the subjective and objective content of the interview. In this case, the resident is suffering from a loss (the pet cat) and she was grieving.

P = Plan content. The "P" contains the actions and interventions to resolve the problem or need identified by the assessment. In this case, the social worker, knowing the loss of a loved pet is difficult, provided several interventions around the issue of grieving:

- social worker to provide several brief visits with the resident over the next 2 weeks;
- social worker to provide the resident with the opportunity to talk about the pet;
- social worker to provide the opportunity to discuss the disposition of the pet's remains;
- social worker to alert other team members about the loss of the pet to engage them in providing support as well.

DO SOCIAL WORKERS ALWAYS WRITE SUCH DETAILED NOTES?

No. Unfortunately, time constraints in nursing facilities rarely allow for such detailed notes in resident visits. However, the SOAP format does provide an excellent outline. Often social workers will provide a detailed identification of a problem or need that the resident is experiencing, but later in the note, the social worker fails to provide the planned intervention or the resolution to the problem. The catchall phrase, *Social service will follow,* unfortunately does not contribute the necessary information to the reader of whether problem(s) will be addressed.

HOW CAN SOCIAL WORKERS PROVIDE
THE INFORMATION?

Some social workers are more skilled at expressing in writing their work with residents. For those who find resident notes difficult, they can use the SOAP format as a basic question and answer model. One sentence for each component will convey the situation in a succinct fashion. For example, our previously discussed resident case could be adequately addressed below:

> *3/13 Mrs. M. appeared sad and teary about the recent death of her beloved pet cat yesterday. (See nursing note of 3/12.) She told this social worker that the cat, Smoky, was 18 years old. It appears that she is grieving this recent loss. Social service will visit several times briefly over the next 2 weeks, provide her with an opportunity to reminisce about the cat and provide support around her grief.*

This note provides the key information, provides a backup in another discipline where the information is also noted, and most importantly, it tells the reader that Mrs. M. is going to have someone help her with her loss through the interventions of the social worker. This note indicates that there is a realistic time frame for the intervention and a follow-up note would be expected following the 2-week intervention.

HOW ARE NOTES OR OTHER MATERIAL
SIGNED IN THE CHART?

All notes, MDS, Care Plans, etc., should be signed by the social worker with his or her state license level. (If the facility is in a specific state where they are utilizing social work designees, the social worker designee should indicate his or her official status following the name.) For example: Jane Brown, LSW. This indicates that Jane Brown is a duly "licensed social worker." It does not indicate her educational background. It is important for the social worker to identify the regulations regarding the status of social workers in the state where they reside.

While educational attainments are important, BSW or MSW or PhD do not necessarily qualify the person to provide social work in the nursing facility. Oftentimes it is only the license that allows social workers to practice the profession of social work in the nursing facility, and that legally validates notes or other documentation.

Students, who are from a college accredited by the National Council of Social Work Education, and serving an internship in the facility, can write notes, but they must be co-signed by the supervising social worker. The role of the student social work intern should be clarified through a facility policy as well.

In states where there is a social service designee, notes are signed as the designee. A social work designee is neither a social worker by license nor by training and should indicate his or her status according to each particular state's guidelines. Social worker designees should obtain appropriate guidelines from his or her state surveyors. The status of the person signing the chart material is clear in this example: Susan James, Social Worker Designee.

WHAT KINDS OF INFORMATION DOES THE SOCIAL WORKER DOCUMENT, OTHER THAN QUARTERLY NOTES?

Social workers should be noting any or all changes in the resident while they are in the facility. This can be quite a daunting task at times. It must be remembered, however, that some residents have few changes, and their charts correspondingly have few notes or interventions. Social workers generally document the following (though there may well be other areas included):

- all presentation of residents rights in the facility;
- all room changes or transfers from one unit to another;
- all plans for discharges and the process for such (meetings with residents, family, community services, etc);
- all mental health changes;
- referrals to psychiatric evaluation or psychiatric team;
- significant physical changes, improvement, or decline;
- changes in advance directives, such as a DNR to a "full resuscitation" or a change in a guardianship or health care proxy agent;
- death of a family member, or significant health problem;
- increases in agitation or hostility;
- facility notices given;
- attainment of goals before care plan meeting;
- financial changes; and/or
- any family meetings.

SHOULD THE SOCIAL WORKER DOCUMENT THE CARE PLAN MEETINGS IN THE SOCIAL SERVICE SECTION OF THE CHART?

This question has a two-tailed answer. Many social workers mix up care plan meetings with social service quarterly notes because they coincide time-wise. The time of the social worker at the care plan meeting is generally spent reviewing the social service or shared goals and interventions to see if the resident has improved or declined. It is this information that should be entered on the chart. If the resident or family member brings up questions at the care plan meeting, it may be appropriate for the social worker to include this information in the quarterly note. This is particularly relevant when the issues or questions pertain to social service. For the social worker to reiterate the interdisciplinary care plan meeting in social service quarterly notes, however, is redundant and not practical. Social service notes should be reserved for documenting the resident's responses to and progress toward the social worker's intervention(s).

SUGGESTED READINGS

Egan, G. (1994). *The skilled helper.* Pacific Grove, CA: Brooks/Cole Publishing Co.

Halley, A. A., Kopp, J., & Austin, M. J. (1998). *Delivering human services: A learning approach to practice.* New York: Longman.

Klenk, R. W., & Ryan, R. M. (1974). *The practice of social work.* Belmont, CA: Wadsworth Publishing Company.

Morales, A. T., & Sheafor, B. W. (1995). *Social work: A profession of many faces.* Boston: Allyn and Bacon.

Scharam, B., & Mandell, B. R. (1994). *An introduction to human services policy and practice.* New York: MacMillian College Publishing Co.

Zuckerman, E. (1995). *Clinician's thesaurus.* New York: The Guilford Press.

CHAPTER SIX

Legal Auspices of Social Work

WHAT ARE THE LAWS REGARDING SOCIAL WORK IN NURSING FACILITIES?

As with may other professions throughout the United States, the respect for the client's need for competent services has driven the legal requirements for social work practice. As the general practice of social work has been licensed in many states, this requirement applies to nursing homes as well.

The social worker functions in the nursing facility under two major governing auspices, state regulations and laws, and federal laws. Many states regulate both the social work in LTC facilities as well as the licensure of all social workers. Both the federal government and the individual states have enacted specific laws that govern the general description of the social worker's qualifications as well as the range of services to be provided to residents in nursing facilities. All social workers should be familiar with the laws regarding their professional positions in the facilities.

WHAT ARE THE SPECIFIC STATE LAWS REGARDING SOCIAL WORK IN NURSING FACILITIES?

Many states have specific laws regarding social work in nursing homes. Some states are very specific about the type of social services expected; others are less demanding. The state of Georgia, for example has mandated social services in nursing homes since 1964. In Massachusetts, Massachusetts General Law (M.G.L.) provided for social services in LTC facilities through

> M.G.L. Section 150.011(E)(4) that stated, "All facilities shall provide sufficient ancillary social service personnel under appropriate supervision to meet the emotional and social needs of the patients or residents."
>
> M.G.L. Section 150.011 (E)(1) further states: "All facilities that provide care for more than 80 patients or residents shall provide a minimum of one halftime social worker. If the social worker is a BA social worker, the facility

shall provide consultation from an MSW social worker for at least 8 hours per month."

Generally these regulations and laws have addressed the need to meet the emotional and psychosocial needs of the residents in the facility as well as options for the facility to arrange for services from an appropriate outside agency.

Social work state licenses indicate a social worker's ability to provide services in a nursing home. In California, there is a requirement of a license for practicing social work, but there are also non-licensed social work designees providing social work in nursing facilities.

WHAT ARE THE ISSUES AROUND DESIGNATING SOCIAL WORK IN NURSING FACILITIES?

The issue of providing social work in nursing homes without training is an issue of concern and controversy. "Nursing home social work can be a lonely, complex, difficult job even for those with education and training. For the untrained, even with occasional consultation from a licensed social worker, the job borders on the impossible, and they can cause more problems than they solve" (O'Neill, 2000, p. 1).

Many states and for multiple reasons have legislated the role of the nursing home social worker to be filled by a "designee." Nursing homes have appealed to state legislatures that the cost of having professionally trained, licensed social workers would be too much and in some cases, there has been a fear that there are not an adequate number of licensed social workers to hire. As a result, nursing homes, even in states where licensing of social workers is present, there is significant assignment of social work duties to a non-licensed staff person. "NASW in November (2000) has signed a formal complaint to the inspector general of the Department of Health and Human Services asserting that nursing homes nationwide are violating federal laws, state laws and federal regulations by allowing 'social services designees' to perform professional social work services in many of the nation's 17,000 nursing homes" (2001, p. 1). The article further states:

> Some of the functions of the nursing home social worker that the complaint says would be beyond the skills of those without social work education and training include
>
> - Implementation and psychosocial interventions for residents with dementia, behavior symptoms, depression, chronic or acute pain, difficulty with personal interactions, legal or financial problems, inability to cope with the loss of function and need for emotional support.
> - Representing the residents' biopsychological and mental health concerns on nursing home interdisciplinary care teams.
> - Complete accurate psychosocial assessments and planning interventions.

- Identifying and assuring delivery of required psychosocial and mental health services. (O'Neill, 2001, p. 1)

In addition, the status of the social work designee is unique in the nursing home. All other professionals with whom the resident and family have contact are licensed, trained, and regulated, e.g., physicians, physician's assistants, nurses, nursing assistants, and physical and occupational therapists.

HOW DOES THE FEDERAL GOVERNMENT REGULATE SOCIAL WORKERS IN NURSING FACILITIES?

The Omnibus Reconciliation Act of 1987 provided for social workers in nursing facilities *Rules and Regulations* (September 1991):

§483.15(g) To assure that sufficient and appropriate social services are provided to meet the resident's needs.
§483.15(g) (1) The facility must provide medically-related social services to attain or maintain the highest practicable physical, mental, and psychosocial well-being of each resident. (2) A facility with more than 120 beds must employ a qualified social worker on a full-time basis. (3) Qualifications of a social worker. A qualified social worker is an individual with:
(i) A bachelor's degree in social work or a bachelor's degree in a human services field including but not limited to sociology, special education, rehabilitation counseling and psychology and
(ii) One year of supervised social work experience in a health care setting working directly with individuals. (p. 383)

ARE THE DUTIES OF THE SOCIAL WORKER OUTLINED BY THESE GOVERNING AGENCIES?

Defining social work services in nursing facilities has not been made particularly clear by governing agencies. OBRA '87 was somewhat specific about a social worker's qualifications to work in a nursing home, but this piece of legislation did not provide a specific outline of duties as, for example provided for nursing assistants. This has left a wide range of roles and duties to be interpreted as social work in nursing homes.

Some states have voluntary representative organizations in long term care, such as Massachusetts Extended Care Federation. This organization provides information and resources to its members. One such publication is *The Survey, Certification, and Enforcement* book. This book provides Federal regulations pertaining to nursing facilities, as well as state operations manuals, and forms used during surveys. In addition there is a section called, "Guidelines to Surveyors." Medically related social services in this publication are described under the "Guidelines to Surveyors" to include the following possible areas.

Medically related social services to assist residents in maintaining or improving their ability to manage their every day physical, mental and psychosocial needs. Services may include:

Making arrangements for obtaining needed adaptive equipment, clothing, personal items;

Maintaining contact with family (with resident's permission) to report on changes in health, current goals, discharge planning, and encouragement to participate in care planning;

Assisting staff to inform residents and those they designate about the resident's health status and health care choices and their ramifications;

Making referrals and obtaining services from outside entities (e.g., talking books, absentee ballots, community wheelchair transportation);

Assisting residents with financial and legal matters (e.g., applying for pensions, referrals to lawyers, referrals to funeral homes for pre-planning arrangements)

Discharge planning services (e.g., helping to place a resident on a waiting list for community congregate living, arranging intake for home care services for residents returning home, assisting with transfer arrangements to other facilities);

Providing or arranging provisions of needed counseling services;

Through the assessment and care planning process, identifying and seeking ways to support residents' individual needs and preferences, customary routines, concerns and choices;

Building relationships between residents and staff and teaching staff how to understand and support residents' individual needs;

Promoting actions by staff that maintain or enhance each resident's dignity in full recognition of each resident's individuality;

Assisting residents to determine how they would like to make decisions about their health care and whether or not they would like anyone else to be involved in those decisions;

Providing options that most meet the physical and emotional needs of each resident;

Providing alternatives to drug therapy or restraints by understanding and communicating to staff why residents act as they do, what they are attempting to communicate and what needs the staff must meet;

Meeting the needs of residents who are grieving; and

Finding options which most meet their physical and emotional needs.

Factors with a potentially negative effect on physical, mental and psychosocial well-being include an unmet need for

- dental/denture care;
- podiatry care;
- eye care;
- hearing services;
- equipment for mobility or assistive eating devices, and
- need for homelike environment, control, dignity, privacy.

Types of conditions to which the facility should respond with social services by staff or referral include

- lack of an effective family/social support system;
- behavioral symptoms;
- a resident with dementia striking out at another resident, in which case the facility should evaluate the resident's behavior; (For example,

a resident may be reenacting an activity he or she used to perform at the same time every day. If that resident senses that another is in the way of his or her reenactment, the resident may strike out at the resident, impeding his or her progress. The facility is responsible for the safety of any potential resident victims which it assesses the circumstances of the resident's behavior.)

- presence of a chronic disabling medical or psychological condition (e.g., multiple sclerosis, chronic obstructive pulmonary disease, Alzheimer's disease, schizophrenia);
- depression;
- chronic or acute pain;
- difficulty with personal interaction and socialization skills;
- presence of legal or financial problems;
- abuse of alcohol or other drugs;
- inability to cope with loss of function;
- need for emotional support;
- changes in family relationships, living arrangements, and/or resident's condition or functioning; and
- a physical or chemical restraint. (Massachusetts Extended Care Federation, 1995)

ARE SOCIAL WORKERS RESPONSIBLE FOR OTHER THINGS IN THE FACILITY NOT NOTED ABOVE?

It is difficult for every nursing facility to be a "cookie cut" of another. Facilities have different demands, resources, and staffing structures. These components can dictate a varied response. However, it remains for the social worker to assess his or her role and utilize professional judgment and social work skills. The following example comes from a small facility where there is only one social worker and few support staff:

The administrator at Sunny Acres assigned the responsibility of obtaining all transportation for the residents to the nursing department. In addition, the business office provided all the financial services necessary for the residents to obtain benefits such as Medicaid and Mass Health, and handled all the issues related to legal matters. The social worker was assigned, by the administrator, to "get the residents the clothing they needed." While the social worker recognized the need for the residents to have proper clothing, the task seemed to be a myriad of tiny time-consuming details. In response to the residents' needs and the assigned task, the social worker developed a unit by unit CNA reporting system to identify the individual resident clothing needs. Further, she coordinated with the business office to generate a monthly report of information regarding the PNA accounts and resident family responsibility. For residents with families, she developed a "clothing letter," as well as follow-up triggers to ensure that residents received necessary items. A local clothing company agreed to come to the facility on a regular basis to measure and present specific costs and later deliver clothing items. This effective system created positive links between the nursing staff, the business office, and the social worker and resulted in the residents receiving their needed clothing. In this case, the social worker became a manager rather than attempting to accomplish the task alone.

Key points in the above example are

- assessing the problem and creating a solution;
- meeting the needs of the residents;
- professional judgment of the social work role in this situation; and
- supporting the system of teamwork to reach a goal.

REFERENCES

Massachusetts Extended Care Federation. *Survey, certification and enforcement. The Long Term Care Survey regulations, forms, procedures, interpretive guidelines.* (Effective 1995, July). Dedham, MA: Author.
Massachusetts General Laws, Chapter 111, section 71 and 105 CMR 150.000-159.000.
Omnibus Reconciliation Act of 1987, P.L. 100-203, §483, 101 Stat. 1330.
O'Neill, J. V. (2000). Least skilled treating neediest patients. [On-line]. Available:
O'Neill, J. (2000). Least skilled treating neediest patients. *NASW News, 45*(4), p. 5.
O'Neill, J. (2001). Nursing home staffing protest signed. *NASW News, 46*(1), p. 6.

CHAPTER SEVEN

Consultation in the Nursing Home

Social work consultation in the nursing home can be an important function to help the social worker with his role. The following section discusses the components of nursing home consultation.

WHO IS AN MSW CONSULTANT?

The social work consultant in a the nursing home holds both a minimum of a Master's degree in social work, and in many states a top clinical social work license indicating both education and experience expertise. For example, in Maryland, the social worker may have either a Certified Social Worker—Clinical License, or a Certified Social Work License; in Massachusetts, a Licensed Independent Clinical Social Worker. In addition, the MSW consultant to a nursing facility should have

- the skill and expertise in the field of geriatrics/gerontology;
- the knowledge and expertise with the regulations that govern nursing facilities;
- the knowledge and skill with psychosocial issues as they relate to elders;
- the flexibility and comfort with multidisciplinary settings;
- the willingness and comfort level to advocate appropriately for the needs of the social worker, the residents, or the families;
- the familiarity with written resources that pertain to nursing home social work;
- the skill and expertise to assist with policy formation; and
- the ability and skill to provide in-services to facility staff.

WHY AND WHEN DO YOU NEED SOCIAL WORK DEPARTMENT CONSULTATION IN A LONG-TERM CARE FACILITY?

Historically, social work consultation was begun to assist the Bachelor's degree level social worker or social work designee with formal social work supervision and resources. There are several reasons for an MSW social work consultant to be in a facility today:

1. Cost: On site, full-time MSW coverage can be costly to the administration in a facility. Generally, Bachelor's degree social workers are generally paid less than those holding Master's degrees.
2. The knowledge and level of expertise of a new facility social worker may be very minimal in the field of gerontology. For this reason, the social worker can utilize the assistance of the consultant.
3. The facility recognizes the benefits from MSW consultation to assist with maintaining the integrity of the social service department.
4. In some states, the MSW supervision in the facility can be applied or utilized for more advanced social work licensing.

It is important to differentiate the formal consultation in the nursing facility from the supervision. National Association of Social Workers' National Council on the Practice of Clinical Social Work (August 1994) has outlined supervision from consultation in 4 ways:

1. Consultation involves a relationship voluntarily entered by both parties wherein the consultant offers his or her best advice that the consultee can either accept or reject.
2. Although the consultation relationship is characterized by adherence to ethical standards, the relationship is not regulated by legal statute.
3. The authority of the consultant is his or her expertise; legal responsibility for the clinical work remains with the consultee.
4. Because of the limitations in authority and voluntary nature of the consultation relationship, consultation does not meet the requirements of many credentialing bodies or insurance companies (p. 2).

During consultation, there may be components that are similar to supervision, resident care issues, for example, where treatment or recommendations are evaluated or recommended. However, generally the consultant is provided with a very limited number of cases. On the other hand, the supervisory relationship, the supervisee provides the information on each case, providing an assessment, diagnosis, and treatment. The supervisor will review these cases with the supervisee, discuss mistakes, and "intrude into the supervisee's work to ensure quality service" (NASW, 1994, p. 2).

WHAT ARE THE BENEFITS OF MSW CONSULTATION?

The overall benefits of MSW consultation range quite widely. The primary benefit for the social worker is to have a resource person with whom to consult for social service department matters. This can range from exploring policy formation around psychosocial issues of the residents, to constructing ways to deal with facility staff issues, to training new social workers.

Generally, consultants review the facility charts as a part of the contract. A focused chart review offers the opportunity to acknowledge the good work of the social worker as well as implement changes to help clarify the social worker's involvement with the resident and the plan of care. Chart reviews should be multipurposed and objective. Suggestions that consultants make from their chart review pertain to coordination of information, follow-up, and clarifications of social worker interventions. These should be viewed as helpful suggestions.

The MSW is the consultant to the facility as well as the social worker. He or she can provide additional focused in-services or other resources to the facility. The consultant can provide visits to residents who are presenting unusual problems.

WHAT SHOULD THE INDIVIDUAL SOCIAL WORKER IN THE FACILITY EXPECT FROM THE MSW CONSULTANT IN THE FACILITY?

Consultation and supervision is a unique mentoring opportunity that should be beneficial for both the social worker as well as for the facility residents. The social worker should expect

- his or her social worker to maintain supervision times in the facility that coordinate with the availability of the facility social worker; e.g., consultation on weekends is generally inappropriate because the social worker is generally not in the nursing home;
- coordination of consultation information with the skills and needs of the social worker and the facility needs;
- that contract outside facility MSW consultation is *not* supervisory, in the sense that the consultant should not be involved with personnel evaluations;
- the consultant to maintain the highest ethical standards of social work and provide the social work and facility with support around this area;
- that while the MSW consultant works with and often on the behalf of the facility social worker, he or she reports to the facility administrator;
- support, reassurance, guidance, empathy, knowledge, good will, and cooperation around issues in the facility.

DO SOCIAL WORKERS HAVE CHOICES OF MSW CONSULTATION?

In some facilities, the social worker can select his or her consultant for the facility. In other situations, the consultant is either already in the facility, or the facility administrator chooses the MSW consultant. Social workers should have the opportunity to work with consultants who can offer the greatest expertise in the long-term care field. If a social worker feels the consultant is not providing assistance, he or she should speak with the administrator and advocate for more helpful consultation.

If there is a personality conflict between the consultant and the social worker, consultation can have only limited benefits. Social workers need to be aware of, and advocate for their own needs, resources, and competencies when looking for or obtaining consultation.

REFERENCE

National Association of Social Workers. (1994). "Guidelines for clinical social work supervision." Washington, DC.

PART THREE

The Nursing Facility

Pre-Admission and Admissions to Nursing Facilities

WHAT IS THE PRE-ADMISSION PROCESS TO THE NURSING FACILITY?

The pre-admission process is primarily developed to examine the scope and range of services of the referred person. Facilities need to be knowledgeable about the needs of the resident, the financial criteria, and the length of stay anticipated. There are several aspects included in this process:

- present place of the potential resident: inpatient at an acute care hospital, rehabilitation hospital, etc.;
- physician orders;
- payment source, insurance coverage, future available funding (backups);
- medical condition(s) requiring continued care;
- rehabilitation potential;
- screening needs, OBRA/PASARR, LTC, etc.;
- discharge plan.

WHO ARE THE STAFF INVOLVED IN THE PRE-ADMISSION PROCESS?

The pre-admission process to the nursing facility can encompass a variety of avenues and methods. Many facilities have directors of admission or screening personnel who visit hospitals, resident homes, or assisted living settings, in order to provide a personal view of the person being referred. In the hospital setting, the chart will be reviewed; the social workers or continuing care representatives will meet and discuss the individual. In the community, the screening may include the visiting nurses, Area Agencies on Aging, or family members. In some cases medical information may be requested from the last hospital stay or other health care provider.

Referrals to these screeners come from a variety of resources, but for Medicare certified facilities, the discharge planner at the hospital is the key referral agent. Many facilities also have admissions coordinators who may also serve as the facility screener but who also market the facility to community agencies and groups. At times, the facility social worker may fill either or both of these roles.

Some facilities have created admission committees that thoroughly review all the referrals. The admission committee may address specific concerns or issues pertaining to a resident's care, mental status, or discharge. Generally the facility is concerned with several aspects: medical conditions that remediate through rehabilitation therapy, secure payment status either through Medicare insurance or private payments, and behavior that will not be problematic in the facility. When the facility is "down beds" (has a decline in their resident census), however, the admissions criteria may change dramatically.

HOW DOES THIS PROCESS WORK
FOR THE RESIDENT?

A potential resident who is a patient in an acute care hospital will usually meet with the hospital-based social worker case manager, or discharge planner. If the patient is unable to participate, the social worker or discharge planner will meet with the family and inform them that the patient should be placed in a nursing home setting. At times, families will talk in advance with the attending physician and make the request for placement, at other times, a home care agency may refuse to provide services if the patient/client is unsafe at home.

There are a number of factors with which a person and their family has to contend in the placement process. These are

- the change of caregiving; and
- the financial costs of a nursing facility placement

New emotional factors may include

- guilt,
- despair and sadness,
- anger,
- relief.

Whether the resident is cognitively aware of his or her surroundings, or very confused, placement in the nursing home is a time for adjustment. Relinquishing the responsibility for caregiving may be particularly hard for the spouse of a resident who has cared for him or her in the home setting.

DO PATIENTS AND FAMILIES HAVE A
CHOICE OF FACILITIES?

The availability of nursing home beds, subacute settings, and even those subacute units within hospitals vary significantly from week to week and quarter to quarter. A family may have numerous choices for placement, or there may be just a few openings. Because of current insurance limitations, however, there is usually a need to resolve a placement decision quickly; the patient faces immediate discharge home or being billed privately for the hospital bed.

Families and/or friends generally tour facilities before the placement. Few patients in the hospital are able to seek placements for themselves. They rely upon family members and friends to determine what facility will be best for their care. When family, friends or guardians are not present; the discharge planner works with the patient to discuss discharge plans and location. He or she will select the facility and arrange for the discharge from the hospital.

If patients or families have a particular preference for a facility, for example, because of the proximity of the nursing home to their home or based on past experience, and there is not an available bed, the discharge planner may recommend discharge to another facility for short-term placement. There the resident can receive care and treatment and ultimately transfer to the facility of choice when a bed becomes available. This is not an uncommon arrangement, though facilities are sometimes reluctant to take a resident for only a week because of the extensive paperwork involved.

HOW DOES THE ADMISSION PROCESS WORK WHEN THE POTENTIAL RESIDENT IS AT HOME?

As with the hospital setting, there is generally a screener from the nursing home or a group of facilities who collects the important medical and financial data. In the case of home or assisted living setting admissions, generally the visiting nurses, or community involved physician, will be the provider of the current medical information. The financial information and other relevant data will oftentimes be collected at the point of admission. When the social worker is involved, it is an excellent opportunity to engage the resident's family in building good rapport, to support care decisions, and ease worries.

DO SOCIAL WORKERS FROM NURSING HOMES SCREEN POTENTIAL RESIDENTS IN THEIR OWN HOMES?

Yes, at times, nursing home social workers can visit potential residents in their homes. The home visit is an excellent way for the social worker to establish a relationship with a potential resident. Home visits can assist the social workers in understanding the needs of the resident and also evaluate the supportive services necessary upon the resident's discharge. It is important and a good opportunity for the social worker to allay the fears about the nursing home placement.

WHAT HAPPENS AT THE TIME OF ADMISSION TO THE NURSING FACILITY?

The admission to the nursing facility is often a time of a resident, family, friend, or guardian feeling overwhelmed. Although the paperwork for admission to a facility is essential for each section addressed, it can be quite cumbersome to the uninitiated. In addition to the packet of information about the facility and the rights and obligations, the resident who is new to the facility is interviewed by numerous facility staff including, but not limited to, the following:

- Nursing staff obtains a medical history, reviews the referral from the transferring agency and provides an initial assessment and physical;
- CNAs help unpack possessions and mark clothing, if family is not available;
- Social workers provide a welcome, address resident's rights, and discuss social service history and perhaps discharge plans;
- Physical therapy/occupational therapy/speech therapy provide evaluations, discuss treatment goals;
- Dietary personnel discuss food preferences and match diet needs;
- Business office may meet with the family or the resident about health insurance cards, or ways that the resident may have to pay for their stay. The business office may also provide information about Patient Personal Needs Accounts and discuss how money can be put into an account in the facility;
- Activities director will meet with the resident and/or the family to discuss previous leisure activities or patterns, and religious pursuits.

This process can be very exhausting for residents as well as their family members. There are numerous names and positions to remember and the amount of information may be overwhelming to everyone. Social workers can provide assistance around this adjustment period by helping obtain concrete services for the resident or family, by remaining available for the resident or family to ask questions and to advocate for the resident as needed.

WHAT IS MEANT BY THE PHRASE "DISCHARGE BEGINS AT ADMISSION"?

All resident admissions to the nursing facilities have an overall plan of care. This plan of care, whether it be rehabilitation for a fractured hip, or care of terminal cancer, or supportive services for a person with advanced Alzheimer's Disease, dictates a response and interventions that, in turn, dictate *discharge timing*. The admission team has generally evaluated all the pertinent criteria before accepting the resident, and this includes discharge plans. This information is written in the clinical chart, and remains a significant part of the MDS and the care plan.

DO THE ADMISSION DISCHARGE PLANS CHANGE?

The discharge plan anticipated at the time of admission may change during the admission due to many circumstances. The resident's ongoing medical condition, his or her insurance benefits, ability to cognitively return to the community setting, home care plans, or availability and/or ability to pay for the facility bed, all impact the length of stay. All of these criteria may affect and change the resident's length of time in the facility. Resident changes that affect the anticipated discharge plan are generally addressed during the routine team meetings and should always communicated with the resident and with the family. If the resident's goals are not being met due to the resident's health, the rehabilitation team may be forced to discharge the resident from services earlier than originally anticipated.

Admissions that take place under Medicare, Prospective Payment System, or other HMO or health insurance coverage also impact a resident's stay in the facility. Social Workers should be aware of the implications of insurance coverage around admission and discharge and the difficulty residents and families have in understanding the intricacies of health insurance payments. Payment for services does not necessarily mean a resident does not need services, nor does it mean the resident no longer needs to have nursing home care.

For example, if Mrs. Jones fails to make expected progress in Medicare certified physical therapy or occupational therapy treatment for her fractured hip and arm because she has Alzheimer's Disease, the team would have to adjust the treatment plan to conform to acceptable Medicare criteria. This information is generally known and plans are addressed within the staff Medicare meeting time, not the routine facility care plan meetings. In our example above, Mrs. Jones and her family would most likely be notified by telephone, by written letter that her skilled days had ended, on a specific date. The nursing facility staff would then provide Mrs. Jones' care without payment from Medicare, perhaps privately paid or under Medicaid (Title XIX). The direct supervision and observation of the Rehabilitation Team would cease at this point.

This information about Medicare benefits is important to transmit within a three-day window. Residents and/or their legal representatives also have the right to appeal the notice of termination of benefits to Medicare. The appeal process allows continuation of therapy treatment(s) until a decision has been made regarding whether Medicare will pay for the ongoing care.

CHAPTER NINE

Screenings for Long-Term Care

The focus of all good care is to determine need. *Long-term care is not an extension of acute care—it is distinctive in its very nature. Because long-term care continues for prolonged periods, it becomes enmeshed in the very fabric of people's lives. Unlike the situation with acute care, where lifestyles may be temporarily disrupted in pursuit of tangible gains in health . . . the predominant strategy in long-term care emphasizes integration of treatment and living. (The Heart of Long-Term Care, 1998)*

WHAT ARE LONG-TERM CARE SCREENINGS?

Screening for long-term care is one way that the federal government and, in particular, the state, attempt to eliminate unnecessary or premature placement of older or disabled people in nursing homes. One focus of these screenings is eligibility or need for nursing facility care. States frequently include sections that address all available community services, and availability of relatives and/ or friends to provide care in noninstitutional settings. Throughout the states, there are agencies, departments, AAAs (Area Agencies on Aging), or home care service offices where LTC screeners review the submitted material.

In Massachusetts, facilities that have in-patient residents applying for Medicaid submit the latest MDS form. At times, additional information will be requested as well, such as the medication sheets, the physician's orders, and/or other ancillary care providers. As opposed to other forms and arrangements, this information is not provided by fax and is sent in the mail to the local offices.

In Connecticut, the Alternative Care Operations (in the Medical Care Operations Division) unit is responsible for waiver programs and alternatives to nursing home care. Specific programs include the Connecticut Home Care Program for elders, Connecticut's "Katie Becket" model waiver, Nursing Facility Preadmission Screening/Annual Resident Review and a Department of Mental Retardation waiver. The unit also performs spousal assessments and level of care determinations, monitors the Institute for Mental diseases and is responsible for the inspection of Care/Psychiatric Hospitals. (State of Connecticut Department of Social Services, 2000)

In Minnesota, the Department of Human Services provides case management services within a county human services department. The focus of the

Department of Human Services is to enable residents to remain in their homes as long as possible. There are three programs listed in helping community residents achieve this goal: Alternative Care Program, Elderly Waiver Program, and Consumer Support Grants Program (Minnesota Department of Human Services, 2001).

WHAT HAPPENS TO THE SCREENING INFORMATION ONCE IT IS GIVEN TO THE LTC SCREENER?

The information collected and submitted is examined by the identified long-term care screening nurses, who decide, based on the facts provided, whether long-term care placement is appropriate. This decision is then passed on to the individuals making the request for placement; this can be the prospective resident, the family, a home care provider, as well as Medicaid, a primary payer for nursing facilities. If there is not adequate information or the criteria is not met (e.g., the person's ailments do not demand the continuous care and support of nursing home staff), the nurse may call or write the facility or the agency person who has submitted the form and request more data. Disapproval of a resident for nursing home care from LTC screening denies Medicaid payment. Generally extensions can be requested from previously qualifying LTC screening while the facility, resident, and family seek an appropriate discharge site.

WHO RECEIVES THEIR DECISION?

After the long-term care screening is approved, the agency sends the decision to the resident, the family, and facility. At times, the long-term care screener will provide a verbal approval. The typical screening approval (in Massachusetts) can grant nursing home stays for either a short-term stay of 30 days, 60 days, 90 days, or long-term, indefinite approval. It is important to recognize that when a short-term approval is given, it is necessary for the facility to review the resident's progress and either submit a new form, or extend the short-term stay with a short-term reassessment form. Update forms need to be submitted to the LTC screeners in the same fashion as the initial form.

WHEN DOES THE SOCIAL WORKER INITIATE LTC SCREENING?

Although the criteria for long-term care screening varies from state to state and changes, at times, within states, it can be generally said that the social worker initiates the LTC screening under the following conditions:

- before the resident is admitted to the facility, if he or she is determined to be financially eligible for Medicaid;

- when any resident is applying for Medicaid in the nursing home, and may expect to remain in the nursing home beyond his Medicare days;
- residents who have been living in the community and who have Medicaid must also have an eligibility screening done before they enter a nursing home for Medicaid to pay for their stay. Medicaid eligibility in the community does not mean the person is automatically covered in a nursing home. Regardless of the financial eligibility, medical criteria must be met for nursing home eligibility. Medicaid will not approve payment for a nursing home resident who does not have a long-term care placement screening;
- when a resident who has been paying privately for his or her stay in the facility will be depleting his or her resources within 3 to 4 months and applying for Medicaid.

WHAT HAPPENS WHEN THE RESIDENT IS FIRST ADMITTED UNDER MEDICARE?

For those patients who are in acute care settings, hospitals are also designated screeners and they can submit their evaluations to long-term care for approval before the resident is admitted to the nursing home. Residents who require longer rehabilitation or treatment generally require another full screening following their Medicare days.

If the resident in the nursing home came into the facility under Medicare Part A and with the express idea that her stay was going to be short, and her recovery does not progress enough to allow her to return to the community, a screening form can be done post-admission. It is important to remember that Medicaid can pay for services 3 months prior to application. The problems with patient paid amounts and untimely payments to the facility, however, are avoided when Medicaid is navigated in a synchronized fashion with the resident's known physical care needs and her existing insurance benefits.

WHAT HAPPENS WHEN A RESIDENT TRANSFERS TO ANOTHER FACILITY?

Although specific detail can vary from state to state, long-term care screening must able be done for any residents transferred to another nursing facility whether this transfer with within or out of state. The nursing home that is transferring is responsible for initiating the screening. The receiving facility must request the screening before accepting the resident and be assured by the long-term care screening nurse that the resident is still eligible for nursing home care. LTC screenings do not have time frames of validity. They are placement specific. Even if a screening is done a week before, it needs to be redone to accommodate a transfer between facilities.

WHAT HAPPENS IF A RESIDENT IS DETERMINED NOT TO NEED LONG-TERM CARE AND DOES NOT HAVE FINANCIAL RESOURCES TO STAY IN THE FACILITY AS A PRIVATE PAY RESIDENT?

There are times when the criteria and the needs of the person being screened do not meet the standards set by the LTC screeners for nursing home placement. Generally, this occurs when the resident has recovered sufficiently from an acute illness and he or she is able to return to the community. Occasionally, the screening is not approved when the person has been in the facility for a long time as a private payer, and needs "conversion" to Medicaid. Discharge to the community is the only alternative at this point.

If long-term care approval is not indefinite, the social worker can request extensions from LTC screening. Generally these can be given in 60-day blocks. It is then up to the social worker to work with the resident, family and community resources to provide non-skilled, alternative housing for the resident. Communication with screeners is very important in providing an accurate picture of a resident's condition. Anticipation of a resident's physical condition at the time of conversion can decrease problems with eligibility.

WHAT ARE OBRA PASARR SCREENINGS?

Subpart C: Pre-admission Screening and Annual Review of Mentally Ill and Mentally Retarded Individuals of the Omnibus Budget Reconciliation Act (OBRA) provided for identification and screening of those potential residents of nursing homes who have diagnoses of mental illness or mental retardation (as diagnosed using the *Diagnostic and Statistical Manual of Mental Disorders*, 3rd edition, revised in 1987). The purpose of this screening process is to evaluate the person's service needs and requirements as well as determine whether nursing home placement is appropriate and what if any specialized services are needed. The screening was designed to rule out the primary diagnosis of Alzheimer's disease or a related disorder. All assessments are provided in person and should be within the OBRA mandated timelines of 7–9 working days since referral. Access to all medical records by the resident and the family is part of this screening process.

Results of the OBRA PASARR Screening are provided to the facility in writing and the possible results are

A. May be admitted to the nursing facility. Nursing facility services are needed; any/all services can be provided by the nursing facility;

B. May be admitted to the nursing facility. Nursing facility services and specialized services are needed. Specialized services to be provided, purchased or arranged by the State;

C. May not be admitted to the nursing facility. Specialized services are needed. Needs cannot be met in a nursing facility setting (e.g., threat to self or others);

D.   May not be admitted to a nursing facility. Nursing facility services not needed. Specialized service not needed. Needs can be met in a less restrictive community setting.

An OBRA pre-screening is required when

1.   there is any new admission to a nursing facility;
2.   the resident has any inpatient psychiatric hospitalization occurrence;
3.   a nursing home resident is discharged to the community and decompensates (mental illness primarily) or mental retardation signs and symptoms increase and coping mechanisms decrease, necessitating a readmission to a nursing facility. At that time, a new Medicaid Level I screening by the home care agency will trigger the PASARR process.

An OBRA pre-screening is not required when

1.   a nursing home resident transfers from one nursing facility to another. The sending facility should include a copy of the most recent OBRA screening with the accompanying paperwork. A re-screening is completed on an annual basis;
2.   a nursing home resident is sent to a hospital for medical reasons. If medically hospitalized residents who have had OBRA assessments are subsequently transferred to a different facility, the receiving facility must contact the previous nursing home or the OBRA offices for a copy of the most recent OBRA. At times, highly sensitive information for residents with diagnoses of Mental Illness or Mental Retardation transmitted by the OBRA screenings. The purpose of communicating this information is to aid in the treatment and care of the individual and by confidentiality is limited to this extent.
3.   a nursing home resident is approved for a 90-day stay and has received an OBRA PASARR screening during that time period. No additional screening will be required if there is a conversion to long-term care nursing status. Screening is required for residents who are admitted to an inpatient psychiatric hospital at or before the 90-day mark.

It is important for all admissions personnel and social workers to examine the admission and discharge process carefully to ensure that they are in compliance with OBRA PASARR screening regulations.

WHAT HAPPENS WHEN AN OBRA PASARR DETERMINES THAT A RESIDENT NO LONGER NEEDS THE SERVICES OF THE NURSING HOME?

If a resident is determined (in an annual review) to no longer need the services of the nursing home or the specialized services of MR (Mental Retardation), MI (Mental Illness) agency, according to OBRA, the state is responsible for

1.   the safe and orderly discharge of the resident from the facility in accordance with §483.12(a); and

2. preparing and orienting the resident for discharge. (OBRA)

The intent of this section (§483.118) of the regulation is to provide some degree of support and responsibility to discharges and cessation of services to residents who reside in the facility.

HOW DOES A SOCIAL WORKER KNOW THE DIFFERENCE BETWEEN THE STATE LONG-TERM SCREENING AND THE OBRA PASARR SCREENINGS?

The state long-term screening is a state-determined arrangement and utilizes a separate design from the PASARR. The state long-term screenings utilize the inpatient MDS and are completed by the nursing facility staff, and/or by other health care providers, such as VNAs and hospitals. The pre-admitting nurse or social worker completes the OBRA/PASARR pre-admission screening form and the actual review of the resident is completed by a separately contracted agency. The nursing facility staff is only involved in initiating the pre-admission OBRA PASARR screening process. It is the specifically designated state agency that completed the process. Generally states have separate mental health and mental retardation authorities. Both systems are designed to review the resident care needs. Both screenings examine the need for care and the facility's ability to meet those needs. Both state systems connect eligibility for nursing home care with payment for care and the timeliness of processing requests is important.

REFERENCES

Kane, R. A., Kane, R. L., & Ladd, R. C. (1998). *The heart of long-term care.* New York: Oxford University Press.

Minnesota Department of Human Services. (2001). *Aging initiative.* [On-line]. Available: http://www.dhs.state.mn.us/agingint/Services/casemgr.htm

Omnibus Budget Reconciliation Act of 1987. P.L. 100-203, 101 Stat 1330 §483.100–§483.136.

State of Connecticut Department of Social Services. (2000). *Replacing welfare with work. The Medical Care Operations Division.* [On-line]. Available: http://www.dss.state.ct.us/divs/medops.htm

CHAPTER TEN

OBRA—The Omnibus Budget Reconciliation Act

WHAT IS OBRA?

OBRA, the Omnibus Budget Reconciliation Act, was a piece of legislation that was passed by the U.S. Congress in 1987. Its primary purpose was to improve the quality of care provided by long-term care facilities and to enhance the quality of life of the residents. The regulations outlined by OBRA were aimed at facilities who participate in Medicare and Medicaid systems of payment, but private, nonparticipating nursing facilities have also been influenced by these new regulations. It is important to note that the passage of OBRA also included funding for states to implement and regulate the process.

The following information is an overview of some of the key points of the legislation. It is relevant for social workers to be very familiar with OBRA and the requirements for nursing facilities because these regulations are a hallmark in residents' rights and access to quality care. Social workers can also utilize regulations for advocacy issues.

Although OBRA was passed in 1987, it was phased into facilities in time segmented provisions, with key years being 1989, 1990, and 1992. This allowed facilities the time to upgrade and to prepare for the changes that these new provisions of the bill demanded. There have also been revisions and amendments to the original OBRA requirements, as recent as October 1, 1999 (OBRA).

WHAT DOES OBRA FOCUS ON?

Highlights of OBRA include Residents Rights in the Nursing Facility such as

- resolution of grievances;
- freedom of visitation;
- notification of changes of room or roommates;
- access to a telephone;

- retention of personal property;
- privacy and confidentiality;
- notification of changes in treatment;
- freedom from verbal, sexual, physical, and mental abuse and from involuntary seclusion.

While some of the above areas may seem simplistic, OBRA's intent was to standardize the nation's many nursing homes. The wide range of services, treatment, and even the description of a "nursing home" vary widely throughout the 50 states. In Texas, for example, a nursing facility is described as being

> an establishment that provides food, shelter, and nursing care for four or more persons who are unrelated to the owner and provides minor treatment under the direction and supervision of a physician, or other services that meet some need beyond the basic provision of food, shelter and laundry. (Texas Department of Human Services, Licensing and Certification, 2000)

WHAT DOES OBRA CONSIDER A "RESTRAINT"?

OBRA also brought in the issue of the use of restraints. Restraints can be either physical or chemical. Physical restraints consist of *anything that interferes with, or restricts a person's decision to move about freely*, e.g., geri-chairs with attached tables, full or partial bed rails, posies, lap belts that the residents cannot loosen themselves, vest restraints, cuff restraints, etc. The focus of these restraints in the past was to prevent residents from falling and causing harm to themselves. Physical restraints were also commonly used to prevent confused residents from disrobing, wandering outside the facility, or going into other residents' rooms. It helped the staff in keeping residents under control. Restraints, at times, could be used to "discipline" an uncooperative resident.

ARE THE RESULTS OF USING RESTRAINTS ALWAYS NEGATIVE?

The results of these physical restraints was to increase the resident's disability and diminish their strength. Resident restraints were supposed to be released every 15 minutes, or at the very longest time, every 2 hours. Unfortunately, the timed releases did not have the positive effect of maintaining the resident's physical and emotional status. In fact, studies and observation indicated that restrained residents actually had greater risks for falls because of their reduced physical mobility! For example, when bed rails were fully extended, residents who were confused or who did not want to wait for assistance to go to the toilet, climbed over or through the bed rails, frequently falling in their efforts to escape. Residents in vest posies, though infrequently, strangled themselves in their exertions to wriggle free.

OBRA has focused on the freedom of movement for residents in nursing facilities to promote better overall health and dignity. Previously confined for hours to table chairs (geri-chairs), wheel chairs, or beds, residents quickly lost muscle tone and increased their risk for more serious health problems. At the same time, the reduction of both physical and chemical restraints has in some cases increased residents' risks for falls because of confusion and/or memory loss. In general, nursing facilities responded to this dilemma by increasing supervised ambulatory time during the day and directing staff to maintain closer observation of residents who are at risk.

WHAT ARE THE WAYS RESTRAINTS HAVE BEEN LESSENED?

Ingenuity and technology have helped to create less restrictive environments. Ambulatory, wandering, confused residents now have bracelet or ankle wander guards that cause buzzers to sound when the identified person attempts to exit a door. Additional technology has made codepad keyed or button door alarms commonplace and allows staff to monitor multiple entrances and exits. Staff, when alerted to a wandering resident, can redirect the person to safer areas of the facility.

For the less mobile residents, there are chair alarms, which, when the resident tries to stand, emit a piercing noise to alert both the staff and the resident. These alarms also help remind the resident not to stand without assistance. The effect of these devices is to support the resident's independence, at the same time providing a reminder not to exit, stand, or leave the bed without assistance.

WHAT IS MEANT BY A "CHEMICAL RESTRAINT"?

Chemical restraints consist of any psychoactive medication that is classified as an antipsychotic. Residents who are in need of antipsychotic medication even when they have a psychiatric diagnosis, are considered to be "chemically restrained." This is a very difficult area because of the numerous disorders, including the dementias and organic conditions that create significant changes in a person's behavior, cognitive functioning, and ability to accept care in an institutional setting. The risks of taking antipsychotic medication are significant, however. Side effects from these medications range from mild, reversible hand tremors, to nonreversible tardive dyskinesia. OBRA targeted these drugs because of their past extensive use in nursing homes and the negative effect that these have had upon older residents. (See also the chapters on Mental Health Consultants and Antipsychotic Medication.)

Protocols have been established for the use of medication that can be administered in a nursing facility that are different from a hospital setting. In fact, the onus and efforts of the long-term care setting are to minimize or eliminate all unnecessary antipsychotic medication that is not being used to treat the resident's medical condition. Reductions (titration down) are generally attempted three times, with close observation of the resident's response. If the resident's symptoms return, the resident can then be placed on the lowest effective dosage, generally permanently. However, the antipsychotic medication is always subject to review by the team, the consulting psychiatrist, and the consulting pharmacist.

WHAT OTHER ASPECTS OF NURSING FACILITY CARE DID OBRA CHANGE?

OBRA provides regulation for nurse aide training (a 75-hour course), testing, registration, and an additional 12 hours of in service training every year. Social work has been also regulated to include "A facility with more than 120 beds must employ a qualified social worker on a full-time basis." OBRA further determines what is a "qualified social worker": "A Bachelor's degree in social work or Bachelor's degree in a human services field including but not limited to sociology, special education, rehabilitation counseling, and psychology. One year of supervised social work experience in a health care setting working directly with individuals," is also included, though OBRA does not specify licenses for social workers. However, all social workers in any state must comply with specific state regulations regarding the practice of social work in the nursing facility. In some cases there are minimum license levels to perform social work in a nursing facility. A number of states have determined the cost of having licensed social workers work in a nursing home is too expensive. Although almost every state has social work licensing, they have determined social work designees may fill the job of a nursing home social worker. For example, the following states have indicated that they allow social work designees: Connecticut, Hawaii, Idaho, Kansas, Missouri, North Carolina, and Tennessee.

In other cases, states have been specific about the level of license a social worker must have in order to work in a nursing home. For example, in Massachusetts the minimum license is the Licensed Social Worker (LSW). The LSWA (Licensed Social Work Assistant) license status is not sufficient to perform social work duties in the facility. *Co-signatures for non-licensed or LSWA status workers are not considered adequate social work coverage by the Department of Public Health.*

Prior to OBRA, nursing homes had attained classifications which individual states designated. Some facilities had been designated as "Skilled Nursing Facilities" or "Intermediate Care Facilities." Now the requirements for licensed nursing staffing in facilities are the same for both and the designations are no longer used, as "nursing facility" has become the ubiquitous, umbrella name. Other designations indicating "level" of care, such as "rest homes" have not been changed.

WHAT DID OBRA HAVE TO DO WITH THE MINIMUM DATA SET?

OBRA is the initiator of the Minimum Data Set, better known as the MDS. Envisioned as the primary tool for analysis of the resident's needs, the goal is to have a comprehensive assessment of the resident within a time frame of no more than 14 days or for Medicare's Prospective Payment System (PPS), a window time frame of a maximum of 8 days from admission (PPS is briefly explained in chapter 14). Quarterly reviews (a shorter version of the initial assessment) are mandatory (minimum of every 90 days), unless there is a significant change in the resident's physical or mental condition. Changes can initiate a complete, fresh assessment. The complete information from the MDS is provided to individual states as well as the federal government. Releases for this are provided in admission information.

Standardization of the quality of care for nursing home residents has been sought through this legislation. Some of these key components promote the notion that residents should have the opportunity "to attain or maintain their highest practicable physical, mental, and psychosocial well-being."

Doris Carnevali (1993) provides a brief outline of some important elements for Activities of Daily Living:

- "The category of activities in daily living includes anything that the individual does as a part of daily living that is relevant to the present health situation. The activities may involve those of the patient as well as others who share that daily living and thus affect the patient. This includes not only caregivers and family members, but also health care workers" (p. 7).
- Mental and Psychological Functioning. OBRA provided the recognition that mental illness and mental retardation required different services at times, and hence developed advanced placement screening. Residents are screened before admission to nursing facilities for the diagnosis of both mental illness and mental retardation. Arrangements for the provision of treatment for any mental and psychological difficulties are the responsibility of the facility.
- Transfer and Discharge. This addresses the movement of the resident within the facility, from the "certified" section of the facility to the "non-certified" section of the same facility. (This issue for the social worker is explored more fully in chapter 11.)
- Pressure Sores. Pressure sores must not develop or must be healed unless the resident's physical condition makes them unavoidable. (Pressure sores quickly develop when a person is immobilized in a bed or chair for long periods of time.)
- Resident Rights. The resident has the right to a dignified existence, self-determination, and communication with and access to persons and services inside and outside the facility. The facility must promote and protect the resident's rights.
- Range of Motion. Range of motion can be loosely defined as the range of physical mobility of the person's limbs and body. The facility must prevent any decrease in the range of motion of residents unless it can be demonstrated that the resident's condition makes such increased limitation unavoidable.

HOW MIGHT THE IMPACT OF OBRA UPON NURSING FACILITIES BE SUMMARIZED?

In summary, the impact that OBRA has had on nursing facilities and the lives of residents is profound. OBRA has decreased the large variations among long-term care facilities across the country as well as increasing similar standards of care for residents. As noted previously, the minimum standards for staffing have been established, and issues of restraints, abuse, and poor care have been addressed. Although OBRA has created an increase in paperwork, the primary outcomes of this sweeping legislation, over the last 10 years, have been to increase the quality of life for residents and sustain their rights as individuals. Social workers are a designated part of this process and they can find support for good social work for residents and their families in this act.

REFERENCES

Carnevali, D. (1993). *Nursing management for the elderly*. Philadelphia: J. B. Lippincott Company.

Licensing and Certification. (2000). Texas Department of Human Services. [On-line]. Available: http://www.dhs.state.tx.us/programs/ltc/certification.html

Omnibus Budget Reconciliation Act of 1987. P.L. 100-203 Stat. 1330 Part 483. Requirements for States and Long Term Care Facilities. Subpart A [Reserved] Subpart G. Requirements for Long Term Care Facilities. Pages 373–433.

CHAPTER ELEVEN

Transfer and Discharge

WHAT IS MEANT BY "DISCHARGE"?

It is important to differentiate between *transfer* and *discharge*. Transfer is moving the resident from the facility to another legally responsible institutional setting. Discharge is moving the resident to a noninstitutional setting when the releasing institution ceases to be responsible for the resident's care.

The rules and regulations regarding admission, transfer and discharge are defined in the Omnibus Budget Reconciliation Act of 1987. These rules and regulations are a part of the nursing home residents' rights. These regulations may be found under §483.12 "Admissions, transfer and discharge rights."

(a) Transfer and discharge
(1) Definition: Transfer and discharge includes movement of a resident to a bed outside of the certified facility whether that bed is in the same physical plan or not. Transfer and discharge does not refer to movement of a resident to a bed within the same certified facility.

WHAT IS THE PURPOSE BEHIND THIS REGULATION?

The purpose of the regulation is to promote the rights of residents to fair and equitable treatment while they are in a nursing facility. This law affirms nursing home residents will not be casually admitted, transferred or discharged without prior notification or without a specific reason.

Schneider and Sar (1998) discuss the importance of relocation and transfers in terms of five ethical components:

1. autonomy and competency,
2. paternalism,
3. duty to do good and avoid harm,
4. obligation to institutions, laws, fiscal limitations and regulations,
5. duty to act fairly and tell the truth. (p. 106)

The nursing facility staff is required to address the issues of admission, transfer and discharge within the framework of the rules and regulations of both state and federal governments. The ethical outline as noted above provides an excellent resource for background and intent.

WHAT ARE THE REASONS A FACILITY CAN TRANSFER OR DISCHARGE A RESIDENT?

OBRA lists five major reasons for discharge; §483.12:

(2) Transfer and discharge requirements. The facility must permit each resident to remain in the facility, and not transfer or discharge the resident from the facility unless—
(i) The transfer or discharge is necessary for the resident's welfare and the resident's needs cannot be met in the facility;
(ii) The transfer or discharge is appropriate because the resident's health has improved sufficiently so the resident no longer needs the services provided by the facility;
(iii) The safety of individuals in the facility is endangered;
(iv) The health of individuals in the facility would otherwise be endangered;
(v) The resident has failed, after reasonable and appropriate notice, to pay (or to have paid under Medicare or Medicaid) for a stay at the facility. For a resident who becomes eligible for Medicaid after admission to the nursing facility, the nursing facility may charge a resident only allowable charges under Medicaid; or
(3) Documentation. When the facility transfers or discharges a resident under any of the circumstances specified in paragraphs (a)(2)(i) through (v) of this section, the resident's clinical record must be documented. The documentation must be made by
(i) The resident's physician when transfer or discharge is necessary under paragraph (a)(2)(i) or paragraph (a)(2)(iv) of this section.

HOW DOES THE SOCIAL WORKER ASSIST WITH TRANSFER AND DISCHARGE?

The social worker has the role of the key discharge planner in most facilities. Transfer and discharge planning can range from helping a resident go to the acute care setting (hospital), to another facility, or to the community. Some of the more important components in the transfer discharge plan are

- resident and family involvement;
- continuation of the plan of care;
- notifications (timely);
- follow-up.

WHAT IS MEANT BY THE TERM "NOTIFICATION"?

Notification simply means that there is a notice (a document) given to the resident or responsible party, that carefully spells out, in language the resident can easily understand, the transfer and discharge policy of the facility, and the transfer and discharge actions taking place. The notice will also include the right to appeal and the process by which the resident can proceed to appeal, e.g., names, addresses, and telephone numbers of public support agencies to call. Notification must be given to all residents in a timely manner, 30 days before the planned move. Residents have the opportunity to refuse.

OBRA, *Vol. 56*, No. 187, §483, further states:

(4) Notice before transfer:
Before a facility transfers or discharges a resident, the facility must—
    (i) Notify the resident and, if known, a family member or legal representative of the resident of the transfer or discharge and the reasons for the move in writing and in a language and manner they understand.
    (ii) Record the reasons in the resident's clinical record; and
    (iii) Include in the notice the items described in paragraph (a)(6) of this section.
(5) Timing of the notice:
    (i) Except when specified in paragraph (a)(5)(ii) of this section, the notice of transfer or discharge required under paragraph (a)(4) of this section must be made by the facility at least 30 days before the resident is transferred or discharged.[1]
    (ii) Notice may be made as soon as practicable before transfer or discharge when
        (A) The safety of the individuals in the facility would be endangered under paragraph (a)(2)(iii) of this section;
        (B) The health of individuals in the facility would be endangered, under paragraph(a)(2)(iv) of this section;
        (C) The resident's health improves sufficiently to allow a more immediate transfer or discharge, under paragraph (a)(2)(i) of this section; or
        (D) An immediate transfer or discharge is required by the resident's urgent medical needs, under paragraph (a)(2)(i) of this section; or
        (E) A resident has not resided in the facility for 30 days.

IS THERE A STANDARD FORM FOR NOTIFICATIONS?

While there is not a standard form for notifications, OBRA regulations state there are certain components that must be included in the *12-point typed* notice of transfer and discharge:

(6) Contents of the notice. The written notice specified in paragraph (a)(4) of this section must include the following:
    (i) The reason for transfer or discharge;

---

[1]In Massachusetts there is 48 hour notification before transfers within the facility, notification of roommates and receiving new roommates.

(ii) The effective date of transfer or discharge;

(iii) The location to which the resident is transferred or discharged;

(iv) A statement that the resident has the right to appeal the action to the State;

(v) The name, address and telephone number of the State Long-Term Care ombudsman;

(vi) For nursing facility residents with developmental disabilities, the mailing address and telephone number of the agency responsible for the protection and advocacy of developmentally disabled individuals established under Part C of the Developmental Disabilities Assistance and Bill of Rights Act; and

(vii) For nursing facility residents who are mentally ill, the mailing address and telephone number of the agency responsible for the protection and advocacy of mentally ill individuals established under the Protection and Advocacy for Mentally Ill Individuals Act.

WHEN DOES THE DISCUSSION OF TRANSFER OR DISCHARGE OCCUR?

The issue of discharge should be addressed at the time of admission. As the social worker addresses the issues around the goals for the resident in the facility placement, discussion of discharge should be included. In some facilities, there are case managers or discharge coordinators who help to plan the discharge of the resident. This does not alleviate the social worker's involvement in the discharge plan or the need for the discharge plan to be discussed with both the resident and the family. The resident/family perception of discharge will have a significant impact upon the rehabilitation gains in the facility.

It is also important for the social worker to help address variant points of view surrounding discharge. For example, some residents may wish to stay a longer period of time in the facility, putting them at odds with insurance payers, case managers, or even family members. The social worker can help both the family and the resident realistically look at the consequences of non-insurance covered "additional time" in the facility or of leaving the facility too early.

The concerns of the resident/family or referring facility should also be examined to help with the plan of care for the resident. For example, if walking up a steep flight of stairs is the stated objective of the resident to return home, how might the rehabilitation team realistically work with this? The social worker might assist with a provision of alternatives. If the plan is uncertain, it is vitally important for the social worker to meet with all members of the team, the resident, and the family to discuss the long-range goals with and for the resident. Not addressing an uncertain discharge plan at appropriate intervals fails to provide the resident with self-determination and an opportunity to "work though" necessary placement or discharge issues.

WHO IS INVOLVED WITH THE TRANSFER OR DISCHARGE PLAN?

The resident, the family, the responsible party or guardian, as well as the entire team, need to work together around the issues of transfer and discharge.

Although this sounds relatively simple, the dynamics of the residents and their families may be complex, and each family member may have a slightly different view of transfer or discharge. Good communication between the family and team about resident's progress toward therapy goals, can improve relationships that are strained. One of the roles of the social worker is to help the therapy team members, the family, and the resident through addressing key issues and refocusing or rearranging presenting goals, if needed.

> The process of relocation brings to light the elderly person's sense of displacement due to disruption and loss of place bonding (Tilson, 1990), and inevitable loss of autonomy or sense of control and freedom to choose how to live out their daily lives. It may also mean an acknowledgement of change in one's health status reminding the person of his or her mortality. (Schneider & Sar, 1998)

IS THE FACILITY RESPONSIBLE FOR PREPARING THE RESIDENT FOR TRANSFERS AND DISCHARGES?

Yes. Orientation for the anticipated discharge is part of the OBRA regulations, but it also is sensitive to residents who need support in making the transition from a setting where there is a great deal of support to a more independent setting. According to OBRA Regulation, *Federal Register, Vol. 56*, No. 187, §483.12(a)(7): "A facility must provide sufficient preparation and orientation to resident to ensure safe and orderly transfer or discharge from the facility."

The preparation for the discharge of the resident can be complicated or relatively easy. The focus of the preparation and orientation for resident transfer and discharge is primarily dependent upon the needs and resources of the resident as well as the assessment of the facility staff. This can be a subjective assessment with objective criteria.

There are also ethical considerations for transfer and discharge. Robert Schneider and Bibhuti K. Sar discuss five factors: "1) autonomy and competency, 2) paternalism, 3) duty to do good and avoid harm, 4) obligation to institutions, laws, fiscal limitations and regulations, 5) duty to act fairly and tell the truth" (1998, p. 115). As the social worker discusses and reviews the transfer/discharge plan with the resident and the family these factors help to clarify the role of the facility team, the role of the social worker, and outcomes for the resident.

HOW DO RESIDENT OR FAMILY ATTITUDES AFFECT TRANSFER AND DISCHARGE PLANNING?

Residents admitted for rehabilitation to the skilled nursing facility are not always clear about their discharge plans. Some may vaguely express they want to return to the community setting. "I want to go home," is not an uncommonly heard statement. The skills and the resources, however, to provide a safe discharge community are also important. It is the responsibility of the team to help negotiate the desires of the resident and the realities of the available resources in community. If transfer to a less restrictive environment is a viable option, then the social worker may work with the residents and their significant others to set up an acceptable, appropriate plan.

> *Mrs. Geraldine Geoffrey, a married 75-year-old woman, was in Yellow Bend Nursing Facility for rehabilitation. Her husband, Fred Geoffrey, 79, had been caring for his wife in their condominium for the past 3 years with the assistance of home health aides. During the last year, the home health aides had been required around the clock. Mrs. Geoffrey was a very heavy woman, confined to a wheel chair, with multiple medical diagnoses including anxiety. Her husband was totally exhausted by his wife's demands. Although he visited every day, his wife would call him at home three or four times a day with a variety of requests. The couple's only child, Amy French, had felt the home situation was unmanageable, because her mother would call her in severe panics whenever her father would leave for small errands. An assisted living setting appeared to be a resolution. The social worker and the daughter reviewed options and selected several options. Mrs. French toured all the facilities and decided upon one, Lark Lane, to show her father. He was somewhat hesitant, but agreed to try this new setting. Mrs. Geoffrey was very uncomfortable in making this decision, however. At first she refused to visit Lark Lane, but later agreed to make one short visit. After several brief visits and a trial "overnight," the couple made the move to Lark Lane, which was a successful transition for both.*

WHAT HAPPENS WHEN RESIDENTS OR FAMILIES REACT NEGATIVELY TOWARD TRANSFER OR DISCHARGE?

Residents and families can have difficulty understanding that they no longer qualify for a stay in the skilled nursing facility. Health insurance carriers, Medicare, and HMOs are increasingly very specific about qualifications for the benefit period. Medicaid recipients and their families, however, are less knowledgeable about the nursing facility screening approvals. Residents and their families can be quite unhappy when they are told that the 60-day period of approved time will not "roll" into a permanent placement, particularly if the family has observed resident confusion or self-care problems in the home setting.

Social workers can help prepare families for Medicaid limitations by discussing the state screening process and how the needs of the resident would be met in the community. Generally either the families or responsible parties and the facility receive a copy of the screening at the same time. (See also Chapter 9, Screenings for Long-Term Care.)

WHAT IS CONTINUITY OF CARE?

Discharge, whether to the community or another setting, represents a change of receiving care for the resident. The discharge plan needs to address how, where, when, and through what agency, the resident will be receiving services when he or she leaves the facility. Every discharge from the facility should be provided with a thoroughly prepared plan of care continuation.

In the cases of acute hospitalization, the care plan at discharge is quite simple, provided with the key basic information about the resident and his or her condition, the resident is "handed over" for immediate attention. On the other hand, a resident who has resided in a LTC/Rehab nursing home for the past 4 months will most likely have multiple community service needs.

Before the discharge date, the resident needs to be informed of the discharge plan date as well as the plans the team is recommending for continuation of care. Services for discharge can be a negotiated process. It is important to tailor the plan to the individual, matching his or her preferences with reasonable, realistic, available services. While it may be advantageous for the person to have a person with them 8–10 hours daily, this may be an unrealistic goal given the constraints of the community service. The home care team will reevaluate all home care issues when the resident returns to the community setting.

All discharge plans should be reconfirmed 24 hours or just before discharge with a follow-up phone call to the agency providing the service. Availability of a service provider can vary and if the service cannot start within a reasonable time frame for the returning resident, then alternative plans need to be in place to help the resident. For example:

Mrs. Suitcase, 79-year-old, childless widow, with severe Chronic Obstructive Pulmonary Disease, was returning to her apartment following a stay at Yellow Bend Nursing Facility. The social worker had originally arranged for her oxygen concentrator to be provided by Ace, Inc. However, in a pre-discharge check with Ace, Inc., it was discovered that they were unable to deliver the necessary equipment for 48 hours because of a trucking problem. The social worker was aware that Mrs. Suitcase needed her oxygen on a continuous basis. He proceeded to call Yup Company, who also provided oxygen concentrators. Yup Co. stated they could provide the equipment the day before the scheduled discharge. A follow-up call to Mrs. Suitcase following her return home confirmed her oxygen services had been started as was planned.

IS IT NECESSARY TO MAKE FOLLOW-UP CALLS TO RESIDENTS WHO ARE DISCHARGED?

It is important to provide some follow-up with residents who are discharged. Generally, the social worker is not responsible for residents once they are discharged, but if service plans have not materialized, it is important for the social worker to contact the appropriate agency and advocate for the former resident. Residents can be quite vulnerable at home and it is vital for coordination of services to take place if they are to remain safe in an independent locale.

Follow-up also provides the social worker with feedback about the success of the services that were offered to the resident while in the facility. Many former residents will give praise and mention their appreciation of the staff following discharge. It serves as positive reinforcement for both the social worker and the staff to hear about former residents who are functioning well following their care. Follow-up notes should be made by the social worker who has helped to close the clinical record as well.

There have been recent changes in home care; Prospective Payment System (PPS) has been in effect in home care since October 1, 2000. This new requirement bases Medicare payment to the home care provider on a specific outcome and assessment service-payment schedule.

WHAT NOTIFICATIONS ARE GIVEN TO RESIDENTS WHO ARE TRANSFERRED TO ACUTE CARE SETTINGS (HOSPITALS) OR GO ON A THERAPEUTIC LEAVE?

Residents who are transferred from the nursing facility to an acute care hospital should receive the same transfer/discharge notice that has been noted above. In addition, the resident needs to have a notice regarding the nursing facility bed-hold policy. *Federal Register, Vol. 56*, No. 187, §483.12(b)(1) stated:

Notice of bed-hold policy and readmission—

(1) Notice before transfer. Before a nursing facility transfers a resident to a hospital or allows a resident to go on therapeutic leave, the nursing facility must provide written information to the resident and a family member or legal representative that specifies:

(i) The duration of the bed-hold policy under the State plan, if any, during which the resident is permitted to return and resume residence in the nursing facility; and

(ii) The nursing policies regarding bed-hold periods, which must be consistent with paragraph (b)(3) of this section, permitting a resident to return.

(2) Bed-hold notice upon transfer. At the time of transfer of a resident for hospitalization or therapeutic leave, a nursing facility must provide to the resident and a family member or legal representative written notice which specifies the duration of the bed-hold policy described in paragraph (b)(1) of this section.

(3) Permitting resident to return to facility. A nursing facility must establish and follow a written policy under which a resident whose hospitalization or therapeutic leave exceeds the bed-hold period under the State plan, is readmitted to the facility immediately upon the first availability of a bed in a semiprivate room if the resident—

(i) Requires the services provided by the facility; and

(ii) Is eligible for Medicaid nursing facility services.

WHO IS REQUIRED TO GIVE TRANSFER/DISCHARGE/BED-HOLD NOTICES TO RESIDENTS, FAMILIES, AND RESPONSIBLE PARTIES?

In this case, the "outcome," that is, the notified resident, is the focus of the regulation. There is no specified discipline in the regulations to provide this information. Each facility has their own process to disseminate information to the residents. Though the social worker may be the identified discharge plan coordinator, however, it is not often that a social service department provides 24-hour coverage in a nursing facility. Residents can and do transfer out of the facility within a 24-hour period.

Since notification of these transfer/discharge/bed-hold rights are a part of OBRA, the law, it would seem logical that all disciplines involved in transfer/discharge share equally in the process. If a resident leaves the facility during "off-hours" then the nursing department is the logical part of the team to provide the transfer/discharge/bed-hold notification. The social service department might provide this material for the balance. Medical records, unit secretaries, or the business office personnel can also adequately provide this information. The important aspect of this process is to inform, notify, and communicate to the resident and/or responsible parties at the time of immediate discharge what rights and responsibilities the transfer entails.

There is no doubt that this can be an area of tension between the social service department and the nursing department in some facilities. The nursing department, as every discipline, is inundated with paper compliance. This deluge of required paperwork can tend to make even patient, kind people cranky. Any compromise between disciplines, however, must keep in mind the outcome of the regulation, that is, timely notification of residents' rights.

REFERENCES

Omnibus Budget Reconciliation Act of 1987. P.L. 100-203 Stat. 1330 Part 483. Requirements for States and Long Term Care Facilities. Subpart A [Reserved] Subpart G. Requirements for Long Term Care Facilities. Pages 373–433.

Schneider, R., & Sar, B. K. (1998). The relocation and transfer of older persons: When decision making combines with ethics. *The Journal of Gerontological Social Work, 30*(3/4), 101–132.

CHAPTER TWELVE

Room Changes

R oom changes comprise some of the biggest issues that social workers seem to face in the nursing facility. Room changes come in the following forms:

- Room change due to a resident's condition that indicates a need for isolation or more observation;
- Room change requested by the resident or family;
- Room change to access a particular section of the facility, such as an Alzheimer's unit;
- Room changes that are *unacceptable,* that is, based on facility administrative need or change in status of payment. (See also Chapter 11, Transfer and Discharge.)

WHY IS CHANGING ROOMS SO COMPLICATED?

Essentially, room occupancy should be dictated and directed by the resident and his or her physical needs for care. OBRA focuses upon this issue to eliminate residents being shifted from room to room to accommodate administrative need or changes in their payment status. However, in today's complex health care setting, room occupancy is far more complicated and this process is connected to licensure and payment systems.

Licensure of the beds in a nursing facility is very important. The vast majority of facilities are licensed to accept Medicaid. In addition to this licensure, many facilities are also contracting a limited number of skilled licensed beds with Medicare (or Subacute) and perhaps with one or several HMO contracts. The licenses for Medicaid and Medicare are separate and designate the type of care as well as payment source for skilled or non-skilled services. Facility beds are frequently dual-licensed with both Medicare and Medicaid. Some beds are triply designated for payment sources: Medicare, Medicaid, and HMOs. In addition, all beds can be paid for privately.

When the term of the resident's stay in the skilled unit ends, either by the person reaching his care plan goals, exhausting his benefits, or failing to reach his rehabilitation goals, the bed payer source reverts to either a private payment or Medicaid status. When this situation arises, the "bed" licensed for either Medicare or an HMO is not being utilized for that particular payment source and therefore the bed is unavailable for any incoming resident who is eligible.

Another issue in any facility is the basic fact that the majority of rooms are not private. Same sex persons share rooms, unless they are a married couple. Often a nursing facility has rooms that include an adjoining, similar size room with a shared bathroom/toilet area between. This means when residents are admitted to the facility, they will be placed with either one, two, or even three other residents of the same sex in the same room.

The administration in a nursing facility may want to move residents for the purposes of "opening up" beds for new residents who qualify for Medicare or an HMO payment source, or to accommodate a new admission of the opposite sex. The pressure to have available beds for new admissions on the rehabilitation unit is quite great, because the skilled unit beds generate a sizable amount of income for the facility.

If a resident moves, after ceasing his or her rehabilitation, to another non-certified part of this facility, this constitutes a transfer/discharge. In order for this move to occur, several elements must be in place:

- the resident must give consent and be willing to make the room change;
- a 30-day notification of transfer/discharge must be given to the resident, their family member, responsible delegate or surrogate;
- the new roommate must be notified (48 hours before the move);
- the transfer/discharge notice must contain:

1. reason for the transfer or discharge;
2. resident rights around discharge and transfer;
3. explanation of the right to appeal to the state;
4. name, address, and phone number of the LTC ombudsman; the agency, name, address, and phone number of those responsible for advocating for the developmentally disabled; and the agency, name, address, and phone number of those responsible for advocating for the mentally ill.

Room changes within the unit can be made within a period of 48 hours. As with any other emergency process, if there is a need for a resident to be isolated, such as infection, a room change can be made immediately. For example, this room change from one non-skilled unit to another non-skilled unit represents many of the good elements that increase happiness and goodwill in a facility:

Mrs. Ryan, daughter of Mrs. Danforth, asked to speak with the Director of Nurses and the social worker at Packwood Nursing Home. At first she was reluctant to address her concerns, but with some encouragement, she spoke of how unhappy her mother was with her present roommate and the unit. "They're nice enough," she said, "but they are so confused. My mother is really more alert than her roommate." Mrs. Danforth's present room was the result of previous unit change and there had been little preparation. The social worker and the Director of Nurses offered another potential unit and room change. Mrs. Ryan agreed to view the room. The social worker provided Mrs. Ryan with a tour of the room and the unit. Shortly after this visit, Mrs. Danforth was taken for a tour of the room with her daughter. They met with the potential new roommate, Mrs. Sommers. The two women shook hands and Mrs. Sommer's introduced her visiting son, James, to both women. Mrs. Sommer's comment, "I'm looking forward to rooming with you. Welcome!" brought a smile to Mrs. Danforth's face. As she walked toward her room, she said she would be ready for the move "any time." A move was scheduled in 2 days. After the move, the social worker checked with both women and the unit staff, who all agreed the move was successful.

HOW CAN A ROOM CHANGE AFFECT A RESIDENT?

Room changes can represent a significant change for residents. Whether it is a simple change of a room within a unit or to a completely different unit, a change for a resident can make a difference. If residents are not out of their rooms a great deal, even the angle of the sunlight coming into a particular window is a familiar component in their lives. Changing roommates, or changing the unit, even with some familiar staff can alter a resident's daily perception of life. Routines, familiar sounds, familiar faces can have a soothing effect upon residents who have poor memories.

Moving a resident who is confused and not cognitively intact is complicated by the way the individual relates to his or her surroundings. If a resident views the world in a limited way through sounds, smells, and the way the light enters a particular room, relocation can have an agitating effect. "Residents' problem behaviors often appear to increase when they were moved, assigned new nursing assistants, or experienced frequent changes in their medications" (Ingersoll-Dayton, Schroepher, & Pryce, 1999, p. 61).

HOW CAN SOCIAL WORKERS HELP WITH ROOM CHANGES?

Social workers can help the facility to become more sensitized to problems of frequent resident moves. Residents who move successfully are more likely to be those who have had some preparation for the event, have had a chance to look at the new unit, meet their proposed roommate, and consent to the change. For example:

Mrs. Lucy Wilkinson, 75, was on a unit where the other residents were very dependent upon the staff. Both the resident and her daughter, Adrianne Bancourt, had been requested to think about a room change to the first floor unit in order to provide Mrs. Wilkinson with a more stimulating atmosphere. A room became available within a week. Mrs. Wilkinson was informed and she asked if Mrs. Bancourt could look at the room. The social worker facilitated the room tours and addressed Mrs. Bancourt's concerns about the nursing staff on the unit. Later, Mrs. Wilkinson and her daughter toured the unit and room, and the two prospective roommates met and greeted each other with pleasant formality, each introducing their family member. Mrs. Agnes Little voiced her welcome of Mrs. Wilkinson to the room and provided a promise to "try to get along." Mrs. Wilkinson accepted the move and decided she wanted to move to the room right away and this was facilitated. The roommates ultimately became good friends.

At the same time when a resident or family member refuses a room change, it is equally important for the social worker and facility to respect this decision. For example:

Mr. Ron Smith, 83, was in Great Pines Nursing Facility. Although he had been in the facility only 10 days, his rehabilitation had only minimally progressed and it appeared that his stay was going to be 3–6 months, if not long-term. The social worker, Mr. Flint, was requested by the administrator to move Mr. Smith to another room and unit so that the facility could fill the bed with a prospective female resident and perhaps another as well. Mr. Smith at first stated that he did not want to move: "I like my room and the view." Mr. Flint, though wanting to respect Mr. Smith's rights, thought the new room might offer a better view and a congenial roommate as well. After some discussion, Mr. Smith finally stated, "I'll do whatever my daughter says." Mr. Flint proceeded to call the daughter, who said, "He's only going to be there a few weeks, go ahead and move him." Mr. Flint made the arrangements/notifications, Mr. Smith signed the facility "transfer" paperwork, and he was moved 48 hours later. A month later, during a survey, Mr. Smith told the surveyor, "That social worker, he made me move. I don't like it here." The surveyor cited the facility for failure to provide the resident with his right to refuse a move.

This move is a typical example of the social worker becoming caught between pleasing the administration and providing residents with their right to remain in a room or move. Social workers need to use their professional judgment in ascertaining whether pressure for a move is necessary or wise.

REFERENCES

Ingersoll-Dayton, B., Schroepher, T., & Pryce, J. (1999). Effectiveness of a solution focused approach for problem behaviors among nursing home residents. *Journal of Gerontological Social Work, 32*(3), 49–64.

Schneider, R., & Sar, B. K. (1998). The relocation and transfer of older persons: When decision making combines with ethics. *Journal of Gerontological Social Work, 30*(3/4), 101–132.

CHAPTER THIRTEEN

Assessment, Goal, and Intervention—The Plan of Care

Planning care for a nursing home resident flows from an interdisciplinary perspective and takes into consideration the resident's past (medical, social, psychological, significant others) as well as the strengths and weaknesses. Nursing facility care plans encompass, in particular, the medical problems of the resident, but the plan of care also includes those issues in which social workers are particularly skilled, the psycho-social and emotional.

Social workers fulfill an important role in the care plan process. They provide the view of the resident from a non-medical, social and emotional perspective. They can help advocate for a resident and or family with team members in the medical system.

WHAT IS THE ASSESSMENT?

Essentially, an assessment, is a tight summary or a succinct view of a resident's presenting strengths and problems or needs. Social workers generally gather information for an assessment from several places:

- interview with the resident;
- interview with the family or responsible party;
- review of accompanying medical information;
- observation of the resident with others;
- observations and assessments of other members of the team.

Assessments are critical evaluations of the person in the environment. The social worker chooses key points in the assessment of the resident to create the problem and need statement. From this point a simple sentence is constructed, for example: *Resident is new to nursing facility, needs to adjust to new routine, staff and roommate.* Many of the problems that are cited in the plan of care are interdisciplinary and require a team response and approach.

Social workers can use a variety of assists in the process of assessing residents. One book, *The Clinician's Thesaurus* (1995), by Edward L. Zuckerman, includes interview questions, mental status evaluation questions and tasks, as well as how to write reports, and lists some psychoactive medications. Another book, *Assessing the Elderly* (1981), by Rosalie A. Kane and Robert L. Kane, addresses specific issues found in long-term care such as: Measures of Physical Functioning in Long-Term Care, Measures of Mental Functioning in Long-Term Care, Measures of Social Functioning in Long-Term Care, and Multidimensional Measures (OARS Instrument, CARE Instrument). Both these books are valuable resources the social worker can use in making clearer assessments both at the time of admission and when the issue of post-discharge care is needed.

DO CARE PLANS INCLUDE STRENGTHS?

The social work assessment should always include the strengths of the resident. These can vary from a resident's ability to verbalize her feelings and insights, to cooperation with care and ability to respond positively to medication. In identifying a resident's strength(s) the social worker can integrate the resident and family participation into the plan of care.

In the institutional setting, the resident's behavior or psychological state is a compensatory response to the problem or need. Indeed the very qualities which may seem to be positively adaptive in a long-term care setting, passivity, compliance to rules, and cooperation, may be less useful in independent community settings. On the other hand, residents with individualistic ideas and fierce independence make more challenging patients. These coping skills are not totally maladaptive or inappropriate, but they may need to have support or redirection to achieve the resident-directed results.

WHAT ARE GOALS?

Goals in a plan of care are quite simply Where the resident's optimum condition/situation should be in a given period of time. Goals should be:

- related directly to the problem or stated need,
- positively stated,
- measurable,
- obtainable.

Pat Gleason-Wynn and Karen Fonville (1993) discuss five types of goals: (1) Improvement goals, describe and project a higher level of physical, psychological or social functioning than the resident is presently capable of. (2) Maintenance goals, directed at keeping residents at their present level of health and functioning and/or slowing the rate of severity of deterioration in their condition. (3) Preventive goals, aimed at preventing complications, either those associated with the problem under treatment or with the approaches or medications used in the management of the problem. (4) Palliative goals, directed at making the resident more comfortable by providing for the reduction of, or temporary relief from, disabling symptoms. (5) Coping goals, directed at help-ing residents understand, accept, develop a positive attitude toward, and/or compensate for their condition or limitation (Gleason-Winn & Fonville, 1993, p. 53).

Goals do not stand alone; they all have an antecedent, or a prior statement. A goal for a person to express that they "feel well for 90 days," therefore, cannot stand alone within the plan of care. An example of a simplistic problem statement would for a person with a "stuffy nose" to have a goal of "clear nasal passages within 24 hours as verbalized and identified by the resident." "Clear nasal passages" relates directly to the problem of a "stuffy nose."

Goals should be positively stated. A resident goal of having "no episodes of hitting over the next 90 days," tends to limit the intervention models to the restraint of the behavior, fails to utilize good problem-solving techniques, and this goal is probably unrealistic. For a resident who strikes out, one has to evaluate the environment and the time periods that surround the "hitting behavior." Is the striking out occurring around personal care? Does the person hit certain staff? Are there any times when the resident does not strike out? Often, asking questions about behavior helps to clarify the problem statement and as a result, this helps to clarify the goal. The goal might be restated as: "Resident will have increased cooperation with bathing/dressing care needs over the next 90 days as identified by nursing assistant observation and daily behavior log." This last sentence then becomes a positive statement of the problem, provides the specific times and places where interventions are needed as well as where the documentation can be found to support the more vague term "cooperation."

Social service goals can be measured in the same pattern. Ms. Penelope Perkins has been uncharacteristically reclusive, mourning the loss of her inde-pendence since coming to the facility. She rarely interacts with staff or other residents. She responds to the social worker's greetings with a brief, stiff "Hello" and does not make eye contact. A social service goal could read: "Resident will engage in increased socialization over the next 90 days as identified by regular meetings with the social worker and developing a positive rapport with the social worker." Social service notes can reflect the meetings, resident behavior, and how the intervention improves the identified behavior.

HOW DO WE MEASURE GOALS?

Measuring goal achievement is often difficult for social workers as they initially work on care plans. For nursing staff, the shrinkage of a decubitus ulcer is photographically clear, as with the physical therapist who can accurately mea-sure the length of the hall the resident can presently ambulate independently. Social workers can measure their goals as well. Residents can and do verbalize their feelings of comfort with roommates; their emotional acceptance, without depression, of placement; or the state of their physical ailments. Interim notes to remind social workers of the progress toward the goals and provide "backups" of the work being done.

HOW DO WE CONSTRUCT GOALS SO THAT
THEY ARE OBTAINABLE?

The old saying, "You can't make a silk purse out of a sow's ear," is also true for care plan goals. Goals have to be reasonable and obtainable, given the problems and needs of each individual resident. While it might be wonderful to change the dysfunctional coping styles of any number of people, the reality is that we often have to accept a modification of the dysfunction. Our goals should reflect potential improvement and positive change, nestled in a realistic construct. Thus, a surly, grumpy resident who argues constantly with all the other residents and criticizes the facility staff, is not likely to become the "poster" resident who speaks highly of the facility and the company. A goal that could be provided in the case illustrated above is, "Resident will express concerns and issues with residents and staff to appropriate facility personnel over the next 90 days." Thus, while the base-line behavior is not necessarily changed, the complaints to anyone within earshot and arguing with bystanders may be lessened with this goal.

WHAT ARE INTERVENTIONS?

Often this is the easiest part of the plan of care for the worker. Interventions are the steps that the social worker takes with the resident to remediate the problem(s) and reach the stated goal. If a resident, for example, has complained of a poor relationship with a roommate and has refused to consider moving to another room, the social worker's interventions might shift from offering a change of room to working with the resident around the dissatisfaction. The social worker could provide individual visits with the residents to discuss developing better communication, or looking for mutually acceptable compromises.

Interventions in the plan of care are the place where social workers can be the most creative, thoughtful, and concrete about their work with residents. At the same time, interventions must be realistic. To say, for example, that the facility social worker will meet with the resident daily over the next 2 weeks is often a difficult or impossible commitment, given the average social worker's schedule. Interventions must be "doable." The plan of intervention needs to be clear, crisp, and match the problem and the goal.

WHAT HAPPENS IF THE PROBLEM
DOESN'T IMPROVE?

There are multiple problems during a resident's stay in the nursing facility, that do not readily remediate. Some problems are "chronic." The important function of the facility's intervention with chronic problems is to evaluate the situation carefully for the best plan of care so that decline or potential harm is minimized. Weight loss with some diseases is inevitable, but facilities minimize the worst aspects of this problem by providing frequent small meals, snacks, and dietary supplements. A confused resident, for example, who disrobes constantly, may not be "cured" of her disinhibition, but with special one piece outfits, her "symptoms" are managed, and she is able to remain clothed in public settings. Our resident care plan should reflect the chronic problems of the resident as well as those that we can improve. For example, some residents have problems with hoarding;

> *Mr. Adams, a 68-year-old, single, formerly homeless man had lived in the Wilbur Nursing Center. He had been living in a two-bed room. His collection of magazines, newspapers, and other reading material was encroaching on his roommate's space. He had also utilized all the floor space under his bed, his closet, and the small chest of drawers. Attempts by everyone to remove his "treasures" were met with extreme anger and hostility. In fact, the last time his room was cleaned, he became so agitated that he had been hospitalized for 48 hours. The social worker, in this case, talked to several people about the problem and a potential resolution. The receptionist's husband had a good relationship with the resident and at times, Mr. Adams would give her husband parts of his collection. An arrangement was devised to provide several large plastic containers for some of the collection and the rest (Mr. Adams's selection) would be "given" to the receptionist's husband to store. This response was acceptable to the resident and resolved the problem for a period of about 2 months. The care plan for the resident included monitoring his collection to prevent an overload in the room.*

In this case, recognition on the part of the facility around Mr. Adams's behavior helped in making a less traumatic resolution. "Hoarding behavior in the elderly represents a complex set of psychological, physical, and sociological factors that require multi-level responses from workers who serve this population" (Thomas, 1997, p. 54). The care plan for Mr. Adams addressed the pressing problem of clearing the room and also addressed the future need to limit the amount of material to the plastic containers. It was the combination of efforts of the social worker, the nursing staff, and the receptionist's husband, that worked together to effect change in this situation.

WHAT HAPPENS WHEN OTHER DISCIPLINES WRITE "SOCIAL SERVICE" ON THE CARE PLAN?

Whenever "social service" appears, the social worker is technically responsible for this intervention or care plan problem. It is important for the social worker to be involved with the care plan process, to acknowledge the social service intervention in the chart, and observe the resident for improvement. If, in the social worker's professional judgment, the intervention is not appropriately designated for social service, then it should be removed from the plan of care. Generally social workers are not inappropriately put on care plans, more commonly they are left off.

CAN SOCIAL WORKERS ADD INTERVENTIONS TO CARE PLANS?

Yes; however, many systems are different. Some systems are computerized and this is technically different than when systems are pen and paper. Most computer systems have points of entry to create additions. Social workers can add to goals or interventions of previously stated care plans.

HOW IMPORTANT ARE CARE PLANS?

Care plans are vital to the total comprehensive picture of the resident. They reflect the outcome of Resident Assessment Instrument (RAI) and serve as the daily tool for working with the resident. Social workers should reflect their care plan objectives in their progress notes and evaluate whether interventions are leading to goal attainment. If after several reviews of the care plan, the goal is not achieved, it is necessary to rewrite it. Although there is not any set rule about the length of a care plan problem and goal, generally every year the care plan should be rewritten if the goal has not been achieved.

REFERENCES

Gleason-Wynn, P., & Fonville, K. (1993). *Social work practice in the nursing home setting: A primer for social workers.* Professional Printing and Publishing, Inc.: LA.

Kane, R. A., & Kane, R. (1981). *Assessing the elderly: A practical guide to measurement.* Lexington Books: MA.

Thomas, N. D. (1997). Hoarding: Eccentricity or pathology: When to intervene. *Journal of Gerontological Social Work, 29*(1), 45–55.

Zuckerman, E. L. (1995). *Clinician's thesaurus.* New York: Guilford Press.

CHAPTER FOURTEEN

The MDS and Social Workers

WHAT IS THE MDS?

OBRA '87 developed the RAI, Resident Assessment Instrument, as a clinical assessment tool consisting of the MDS, or the Minimum Data Set, and the corresponding problem-focused Resident Assessment Protocols (RAPs). The notion was to provide a standard of base-line information about residents in nursing homes. Its implementation and use is nationwide. The RAI, though inclusive of all disciplines, is under the Registered Nurse Assessment Coordinator signature. The RAI is the foundation for the plan of care for the resident as well as the basis of payment for those residents who are under Medicare payment benefits, as of January 1, 1999.

RAI must be completed for all patients residing in a nursing facility longer that 14 days, including

- all residents in Medicare (Title 18) or Medicaid (Title 19) programs in nursing facilities;
- hospice patients when the Skill Nursing Facility/NF is the hospice patient's residence for purposes of the hospice benefit;
- short-term stay or respite patients;
- special populations (pediatric, psychiatric).

A RAI must be completed for a Medicare-eligible PPS resident even if he does not stay the full 14 days. The facility is reimbursed upon the Day 8 and Day 14 assessments and the resultant RUG III classification.

The MDS comes in two formats, Version 2.0, that is, the "long" version, comprised of nine pages, and the "short" version, comprised of four pages. The long version is used under the following circumstances:

- new admission to the LTC facility;
- while under the Medicare PPS provisions;
- significant change in status;
- readmissions to the facility;
- annual review.

The short version is used for quarterly reviews, 90-day intervals, for as long as the resident is in the facility. This shorter version is what is called a subset of items listed on the full MDS.

HOW IS THE MDS SET UP?

The MDS is divided into sections that correspond to letters of the alphabet. Within the sections, information about the resident is logged, answering specific questions. Certain sections are generally reserved for specific disciplines. The assignment of different parts of the MDS to different disciplines is as varied as the names of facilities. Each facility determines the discipline to complete a specific area of the MDS.

Each section of the MDS requests observation for certain time periods, for example, Section AC. Customary Routine, asks for information about a resident, "in the year prior to the date of entry into the nursing home, or the year last in community if now being admitted from another nursing home" (MDS 2.0 September 2000).

Other sections of the MDS ask for information over the past 90 days or since admission. It is important for the team member who is completing the MDS to carefully evaluate the information over the time period being requested and to use professional judgment. This helps to make the MDS information more accurate and the care plan more appropriate to the resident's needs.

WHAT SECTIONS OF THE MDS DO SOCIAL WORKERS COMPLETE?

There is not any particular regulation regarding who fills out what sections in the MDS except a Registered Nurse must sign-off for the entire form. It is, however, logical to have the discipline with the particular expertise responsible for the specialized sections and each facility makes that determination. Social workers can participate in the following sections:

- AA. Identification information;
- AB. Demographic Information;
- AC. Customary Routine;
- AD. Face Sheet Signatures;
- A. Identification and Background Information;
- B. Cognitive Patterns;
- E. Mood and Behavior Patterns;
- F. Psychosocial Well-Being;
- P. Special Treatments and Procedures (1, a, m–q and 1, b, e) (2, a–f);
- Q. Discharge Potential and Over-All Status;
- R. Assessment Information.

Social workers, when they have completed the aforementioned sections of the MDS are also responsible for the triggered RAPs. Care Plans that follow the RAPs are also included in the process.

WHAT IS THE TRIGGER LEGEND?

The Trigger Legend on the printed form follows the response, and is often highlighted in red on original or working forms. *The triggers do not generally show on computer-generated MDS forms.* When there is a trigger indicator, this means that the resident condition, behavior, etc., has a need for staff intervention and the resident is at risk for specific functional problems. For example:

> *Since her admission four weeks ago, Ms. Mimi Roe has been continuously verbally disrespectful to staff (she uses foul language to aides providing her personal care). She complains constantly about the food, regardless of what is offered, and she is particularly uncooperative with certain key staff members. The chart supports this behavior in social service notes, nursing notes and physical therapy notes.*

The person completing the F2. section of the MDS will most likely check the box next to "covert/open conflict with or repeated criticism of staff"; this will "trigger" on the MDS.

WHAT HAPPENS WHEN THERE IS A "TRIGGER"?

The triggers indicate the need for a RAP, Resident Assessment Protocol. This is a written tool that addresses the responses from the MDS, and helps the team member completing the MDS to evaluate further the problem and the responses to the problem. In our example of Ms. Roe, the trigger indicates a "problem" the staff probably needs to address in the plan of care.

HOW DOES A RAP GATHER INFORMATION?

RAPs ask for specific information from the team member. Some of the initial questions inquire about the "nature of the condition, both objective (factual data) and subjective complaints." The focus of the RAP is to determine the complications and the risk factors for the resident who is having the problem/condition/need. The analysis asks for the team member to determine what other services the resident requires to resolve the difficulty. Lastly, the tool examines the resident's strengths, weaknesses, and preferences included in the evaluation.

While the resident has been in the facility, numerous disciplines have had contact with him or her. These observations and direct contact are noted in the chart and form the basis for the identification of both conditions, problems, and the interventions. Logs for behavior problems and notes from all disciplines can be used to verify the condition. Based upon all this information recorded on the RAP, the team member will decide whether to create a care plan for the triggered item. There is a choice at this juncture, not to make a care plan, but the reason must be substantiated in the RAP and based upon whether the triggered condition affects the resident's functional status or well-being.

RAPs are reviewed within the care plan process and the team can alter the plan of care to meet the resident's responses, or continue the plan, or address it as being resolved. Resolved issues are noted in the clinical record, providing backups for the decision.

WHAT HAPPENS TO ALL THIS MDS INFORMATION?

The MDS information remains a focus for the resident care plan in the facility. It is also provided to government agencies, such as the Department of Health Care Quality in Massachusetts. Information from every facility across the nation is generally filed on a weekly basis with their area offices, chiefly Departments of Public Health (DPH). Many facilities file more frequently in an effort to minimize errors. These DPH office sites serve as a clearinghouse for the information that is then provided to the federal government.

Residents and family members should be made aware that all the information provided in the MDS is ultimately transmitted to the federal government. Generally this is discussed during the admissions process.

HOW DOES ALL THIS INFORMATION COORDINATE (THE MDS, THE RAP, THE CARE PLAN, AND THE SOCIAL SERVICE NOTES)?

All the information in the chart should interconnect. The assessments and observations of the resident should be the basis for answering the sections in the MDS. The RAP represents the collection of data, and sets up the plan of care to address the problem(s). All progress notes, social service included, should address the issues presented in the care plan in a succinct manner. It is important that these notes provide the specifics that relate to the total RAI.

HOW DOES THE MEDICARE PPS EFFECT THE SOCIAL WORKER'S DOCUMENTATION?

If the RAI, MDS tool reviews the resident during the PPS period of admission (5 days, 14 days, 30 days, and 60 days), the social worker's notes for sections completed in the MDS need to be supported by progress notes. For example, if a social worker has completed section F2b. and the resident RAP triggers a care plan for being "unhappy with the roommate," the social worker will need to document how the issue is being addressed. If the situation changes within the time frame of the next MDS, this would also be noted in the social service notes and subsequently answered differently on the next MDS review.

PPS does change the response of the social worker's documentation, requiring more observations, clearer interventions, and resident responses. The time between notes is also altered to reflect the specific social work intervention(s). It is important for the social worker to discuss any specific documentation questions with the MDS facility coordinator.

SOME OF THE QUESTIONS ON THE MDS DO NOT "TRIGGER"; DOES THIS MEAN THERE IS NOT A RAP OR A CARE PLAN?

No. The items on the MDS that trigger must have a response, a RAP, and most likely a plan of care. If there is a condition, problem, or need to which the social worker is responding on the MDS that is not an automatic trigger, however, such as "recent loss of a close family member/friend," it should be "care planned." A RAP can be written to formulate the issue and the response of the social worker. The MDS is only the basic foundation for interventions. All disciplines are free—and encouraged—to care plan any additional provisions of care they are making for the resident.

HOW CAN SOCIAL WORKERS LEARN MORE ABOUT THE RAI, MDS, PPS, AND RAPS?

Many facilities have MDS coordinators who have the sole job of coordinating the MDS for the facility. It is very important for the facility to be skilled at completing the information on the MDS in a timely manner because of the payment process. The only responsibility that the social workers have to this end is to complete their particular MDS sections.

The MDS coordinator can provide volumes of information about the RAI. All facilities will have MDS manuals for use with the MDS. There are interpretations for some of the questions and these are frequently discussed in "help books" in the facility. Nursing facilities have focused training sessions to increase participation and understanding of the MDS and RAPS. Other facilities will send interested workers to scheduled local workshops.

REFERENCE

Minimum Data Set (MDS) Version 2.0. For Nursing Home Resident Assessment and Care Screening. September 2000.

CHAPTER FIFTEEN

The Interdisciplinary Meeting

WHAT IS THE INTERDISCIPLINARY MEETING? WHAT IS DONE AT THE MEETING?

The interdisciplinary meeting is basically the time when the team as a whole is gathered together to review the plan of care for the resident. Generally scheduled according to the dictates of the MDS, these meetings are planned around a resident's admission, the Medicare dictated time schedule (see the MDS), or a significant change in the resident's health, or every 90 days past the resident's Medicare days. Generally the nursing staff—an MDS Nurse or Assistant Director of Nurses—takes the responsibility for selecting the resident review time schedule. In some facilities, the social worker may log in these time frames. Most facilities have specific days and times set aside for team care plan meetings. The team is generally given a list of residents before the meeting and it is assumed that all come to the meeting prepared to discuss the residents' current situations.

WHAT IS THE FOCUS OF THE MEETING?

The major focus of the meeting is to review and discuss the results of the MDS, the resulting triggered responses, and to review the resident's individualized plan of care.

The designated RN signs off on the MDS as well as representatives of all the other disciplines that have filled out individual sections. The meeting itself can include all the disciplines: Physical Therapy, Occupational Therapy, Speech, Dietary, Recreational Therapy, Social Service, and the resident or her designated representative.

The members of the team address the problems or needs, the goals, and the interventions provided by the facility for the resident. Depending upon the facility and the members of the team, these care plan meetings can be very brief, or they can be quite lengthy. Generally families/or residents who have special problems or requests are encouraged to select another time for a more in-depth meeting as the care plan meeting generally includes six to ten residents who have a similar review date.

The meeting can also utilize this time to review the chart and update information about the resident's wishes. For example, the wishes of the resident around advance directives or the status of a temporary guardianship could be included.

WHO COMES TO THE INTERDISCIPLINARY MEETINGS?

The team meeting is not an isolated, internal function. Both the residents and their designated responsible party should be invited to attend on a routine basis. Generally notices of meetings are sent to the designated responsible party. The charge nurse, the social worker or the activities director can invite residents. Residents are sometimes shy in attending these meetings and need support and encouragement to join the group.

Attendance at these meetings affords the opportunity for the resident and his family member/responsible party to participate in the plan of care. They have the chance to ask questions of the team regarding the facility's care and to bring up concerns. It should be an empowering meeting for the participants.

Some family members who are uncomfortable with the setting or have a particular area of concern, ask the facility ombudsman to participate. Participants in the care plan meeting should either have a direct role in the facility's provision of service or be a designated representative of the resident.

The dilemma of who sends out the meeting notices can be an issue in many facilities. Where possible, this should be a shared duty between all disciplines and clerical staff. In some facilities there is a dearth of clerical staff and this makes assigning the task of invitations difficult. It is important, however, for the social worker to advocate for his role within the scope of the team. Creative problem-solving for this task can be essential (e.g., families can self-address envelopes for future use, computer labels can be of assistance, utilizing volunteers in appropriate circumstances can help).

HOW IS CONFIDENTIALITY MAINTAINED IN THE INTERDISCIPLINARY MEETING?

The care plan meeting is bound by the same confidentiality rules as other aspects of a resident's care in the facility. The meetings, to ensure privacy, should take place in an area that is separate from the nursing station and the main resident living areas. Doors to the meeting room should remain shut during a meeting. Other residents should not be permitted in the room or within hearing distance of a care plan meeting.

Family members who are waiting for their meeting should be encouraged to wait at a discreet distance. If the resident or designated family member has invited another person to attend the meeting, it is appropriate to address the confidentiality of the meeting.

The written record of the interdisciplinary meeting, regardless of how general or detailed, is generally placed in the chart and becomes part of the clinical record, which is confidential.

ARE THERE SOME SPECIFIC ROLES IN THE INTERDISCIPLINARY MEETING FOR THE SOCIAL WORKER?

As with many other aspects of social work in the nursing home, the role of the social worker at the care plan meeting can be an ancillary position, or the social worker can be the team leader. Some activities in which the social worker may be included are

- preparing for the care plan meeting (e.g., gathering knowledge of the resident and the current case issues);
- providing advocacy for the resident/family as needed;
- assisting the resident/family member to interpret and understand the medical interventions and plan of care presented;
- providing alternative problem-solving or support to team members as needed;
- identifying areas of problems/solutions that the team can address;
- providing additional information of community or facility resources for resident, family, or team;
- providing progress notes in the chart regarding the progress of the resident toward the goals outlined in the plan of care.

In addition, the social worker should be prepared and able to provide mediation for any issues that arise around problems with care between the resident/family and staff. The social worker can prepare the team and/or the family to discuss key points of care and provide a time when, if needed, the resident/family can have a follow-up meeting.

It is important for the team to remember that their medical terminology is not always familiar to residents or their family members. Care plans should be presented in a manner that is understood by all. For example, a nurse reading a care plan verbatim might say, "Alterations in nutritional status with secondary weight loss." The team, when the resident or family member is attending the meeting, should help to translate this statement to "John has had difficulty with his appetite since his last illness, and has lost some weight." Once this has been addressed with the resident and/or family, the team provides a goal and a resolution to the problem. Occasionally, the family or resident can initiate other areas of possible intervention for the team or they can acknowledge with satisfaction what the team is doing to remediate the problem.

The social worker can provide the climate of acceptance and validation for the resident and the family in the initial admission meeting. Throughout the resident's stay, the social worker can encourage care plan meeting participation. It is through empowering the resident/ family member to contribute to the plan of care, that discourse and trust emerge around the resident's stay in the facility. Even when there are difficulties with residents and/or families, open communication about the plan of care creates the most successful dialogue among the participants. For example:

Mrs. Pentel, a 79-year-old, childless widow had been at Settler's Bend Nursing Facility for 2 months. The initial goals at admission had identified the need to ambulate, perform her personal care needs independently or with minimal assistance, and return to her home with greatest amount of home help available. However, by the third care plan meeting, it was apparent that these goals needed to be significantly modified to meet her level of motivation and functional capacity. The rehabilitation team members, occupational therapy, and physical therapy, reported her irregular participation in therapy sessions and her little interest in ambulating, except to get to her chair to sit and watch TV. Her family reported that she had exhibited similar behavior at her home for over a year. The nieces were fearful of her returning to her home because of her lack of safety and self-motivation. At the team meeting, Mrs. Pentel stated that she was content in the nursing facility, and said, "But I know I should go home, but I don't walk good enough yet. I'll go home in a while." The social worker, at the team meeting, explored with the resident her conflicted desire to return to her home. It appeared Mrs. Pentel was not ready to accept permanent placement. A care plan for discharge, suggested by the social worker, changed the discharge plan date to "indefinite" and the community discharge would be based on Mrs. Pentel's activities of daily living (ADLs) competency and ambulating ability. Mrs. Pentel agreed readily to this plan, expressing relief at not having to conform to a deadline.

The social worker in this case advocated for the resident. This compromise allowed the resident to participate in the potential for discharge, if she should increase her motivation and performance, but eliminated the emotionally laden pressure of a specific date.

WHAT FACILITY DOCUMENTATION IS NEEDED FOR THE INTERDISCIPLINARY MEETINGS?

Each meeting is generally documented in the resident's chart. The notes for the meeting are not standardized. Many facilities, however, have a record of the professional staff in attendance, the resident and family member or any other representative present sign a log indicating presence at a meeting.

Some facilities have the social worker function as the "meeting secretary." In these cases, there is generally a form for the meeting, an outline of what was discussed, and overall medical and social changes that have occurred for the resident. There may be check-off sections for standard components of the meeting such as review of advance directives, or permissions for flu shots. These notes are frequently kept next to the MDS and support care planning decisions. The interdisciplinary meeting note does not replace social service progress notes about the resident.

CHAPTER SIXTEEN

In-Services for Facility Staff

WHAT IS AN IN-SERVICE?

An in-service is a program presented within the facility to the staff. These programs represent a wide range of topics and presentation styles, from videos to outside speakers to staff members, selectively chosen to share special knowledge or information. Some topics are very specific for a discipline; an in-service on decubitus ulcer treatment, for instance, would apply to the nursing department. Other programs are more general, for example, facility infection control.

Facilities plan their in-services throughout the month. These are generally scheduled with the facility Staff Development Coordinator who also monitors the timeliness of the mandatory in-services.

WHAT ARE SOME OF THE COMPONENTS OF AN IN-SERVICE?

The following outline example describes a typical in-service:

To establish the group in a comfortable position, it is always helpful to have all group members introduce themselves and their role/job in the facility. Even if the speaker/group leader is a staff member, it is always good to explain their role and their educational background to the audience.

I.   Introduction to Abuse, Neglect, and Mistreatment
    A.   Defining the differences of Abuse, Neglect, and Mistreatment
    B.   How it relates to care of the residents
II. Explain the facility policy for reporting Abuse, Neglect, and Mistreatment
    A.   Using two vignettes as a handout
        1.   Discussion/work in small groups
        2.   Questions & answers
III. Provide a brief multiple choice post-test for the group

    A.   Summarizing knowledge obtained through the in-service

    B.   Reinforce information for use on the job

HOW MANY IN-SERVICES DOES A SOCIAL WORKER TYPICALLY HAVE TO PRESENT?

The actual number of in-services the social worker may do in a facility can very significantly from facility to facility. In some settings, the social worker may only present two or three in-services a year. In another facility, a weekly in-service component is expected.

The type of in-service that is offered often dictates the frequency, for instance, the Abuse, Neglect, and Mistreatment in-service may be given as a refresher to Certified Nursing Assistants (CNAs) and staff once a year (all three shifts). On the other hand, if the Staff Development Coordinator wishes to incorporate the role of social service in orientation of staff, the social worker could be providing this component as frequently as once a week.

If a nursing facility has been cited for deficiencies in the area of residents' rights or dignity or quality of life, the social worker may be called upon to provide more in-services to the staff as a part of the plan of correction.

HOW CAN A SOCIAL WORKER PREPARE FOR AN IN-SERVICE?

In preparation for an in-service, the social worker needs to keep in mind the focus of the program. While there may be a great deal of information about the topic, and the social worker may be tempted to provide volumes to the staff, she should keep the program brief and focused. In-service presentations are generally no longer than 30 minutes. Presenters should make one or two major points and a conclusion that the audience can apply in their work with residents. In-services can be repeated in the original form. In addition, they can have subsequent component parts to provide more information at a later date.

Resources for the in-service can come from a variety of agencies and organizations. If the social worker wishes to provide written material to the audience, she should make sure that it is in language and style that the staff will understand. Journal articles from professional magazines generally are not interesting reading for CNAs. On the other hand, a brief summary of the article, or key points highlighted, can help reinforce important facts for the group. Written material can be provided in the form of a handout or presented in Powerpoint or overheads.

WHAT IS THE BEST WAY TO PRESENT THE MATERIAL?

The best way to present the material is to make it pertinent to the group's interests and fun. Lecture presentations are objective, requiring a sophistication and long attention span. Active participation of the group is a good way to incorporate a variety of learning styles, such as linguistic, auditory, or kinesics. The utilization of role-plays, simple games, and catchphrases can engage the audience. Case studies with pertinent questions for group response are another effective way to present material. Remember also, positive feedback for each participant will help engage the learning process.

Most of the material presented in an in-service is important in staff interaction with residents. In essence this means the staff must *apply* the knowledge, facts, techniques, and rules in different ways. Questions for the in-service process can include;

> How would you use . . . ?
>
> What examples can you find to . . . ?
>
> What approach would you use to . . . ?
>
> How would you solve (the problem) using what you've learned here?

It is also important to keep in mind that changes in either staff or resident behavior are not instantaneous. As social workers, we know learning takes place in incremental stages. Practice of new techniques or ideas and regular in-service presentations can help in channeling new, more effective interactions with residents.

WHAT ARE SOME INTERESTING TOPICS FOR IN-SERVICES?

Topics that are of interest to the nursing staff and the CNAs are generally those that deal with issues or behaviors of a resident or family. Many diseases have particular behavioral symptoms that can cause difficulty with interpersonal relationships and, in particular, caregiving. An in-service on Parkinson's Disease, for example, could help both the CNAs and the nurses examine some of the changes that occur during the course of the illness.

Social workers can observe some of the particular issues on a unit or in a facility with which the staff has to deal. In-services can be planned to meet these needs. For example, holidays can be stressful for everyone. An in-service around caregiver stress can help the staff prepare for their own emotional issues and needs as well as for those of the residents and families.

Although many staff have worked in nursing facilities, many have never had a formal course on aging. The following are some topics for in-services:

- Normal Aging
- Problem Behaviors and Solutions
- Memory Loss
- Abuse, Neglect, and Mistreatment
- Families of Residents
- Transition From Community to Nursing Home
- Death and Dying
- Confidentiality
- Depression
- Sexuality

- LTC Ombudsman Program
- Ethnicity (particular group represented in the nursing home)
- The Role of the Social Worker

All of this information helps to create greater understanding of the role with elders in nursing facilities. In-services are one way to help staff become more sensitive to their caregiving role and their impact upon residents. Education gives new awareness and understandings, creating more effective workers who look for solutions to problems with resident behavior. The nursing home social work role can be pivotal in this process.

DOES POOR ATTENDANCE AT AN IN-SERVICE MEAN THAT THE SUBJECT IS UNIMPORTANT?

No. Poor attendance at an in-service may indicate the staff has not had the opportunity to take a break from their duties of caring for residents. If the units are short on staff, or there have been multiple admissions to the facility on that particular day, staff will not be present for an in-service. If possible, the in-service should be rescheduled for another date.

The social worker can also work closely with the Staff Development Coordinator to set up a time that would be most available for staff. Creativity for times and places helps increase attendance. Banazak and colleagues noted that there is some restrictiveness to staff participation in educational programs: "Barriers include mixed messages about patient care, high turnover and the 'outsider' phenomenon" (2000, p. 69). These barriers can result in lower staff turnout for programs.

Sometimes, the social worker can provide in-services on the facility unit, making the process easier. Providing shift in-services also helps. For example, a social worker might return to the facility for the evening shift, or begin early one morning to accommodate the 11 PM to 7 AM shifts. Staff, generally, will not attend in-services that are not mandatory during their off-hours.

The social worker's efforts to arrange in-service meetings and include all members of the facility team are important in the process of gaining "visibility." As the staff becomes more familiar with the social worker as a part of the team, regardless of the shift, communication can increase about the progress of residents. Thus the educational programs can serve both as a way for the social worker to increase the knowledge and skills of the staff, and also to increase his personal contact and role modeling with nursing assistants and nurses.

WHAT WILL THE FUTURE BRING TO IN-SERVICE TRAINING?

Many facilities have utilized technology to support the needs of the facility and staff. Videotaping, utilizing Powerpoint, and using voice recordings during in-services are a few ways the staff can participate more actively. In the very near future, there may be in-service training available on-line. The learning styles of the staff will be assisted by these new forms of education and training, and this has the potential to translate into increased skills in caring for residents.

WHAT ARE SOME RESOURCES FOR IN-SERVICE TRAINING?

The following is a brief list of resources that can be used either to enhance the social worker's own knowledge or to assist in-service training:

Videos and Movies:

Growing Old in a New Age—13 one-hour programs. Website: http://www.learner.org/catalog/humanbehav/goseries/

Both of the films below are available through Terra Nova Films, Inc., 9848 S. Winchester Ave., Chicago, IL 60643 (773) 881-8491 or (800) 779-8491.

Alzheimer's: A Multicultural Perspective (34 minutes)

Just to Have a Peaceful Life (10 minutes)—Training tool for illustrating the relationship between elder abuse and domestic violence.

Instruments:

Palmore, E. B. (1988). *Facts on aging quiz* (2nd ed.). New York: Springer Publishing.

A Mental Status Exam for Dementia (MMSE)—Available through the Behavioral Science Media Lab, Neuropsychiatric Institute and Hospital at U.C.L.A., 760 Westwood Plaza, Los Angeles, CA, 90024-1759.

Knox, V. J., Gekoski, W. L., & Kelly, L. E. (1995). The aged inventory. *International Journal of Aging and Human Development, 40*(1), 31–55.—Measures stereotypes/attitudes toward older adults.

Other Resources:

Patient Self-Determination Act 1990.

Interdisciplinary Team Training Resource Center—Curriculum products, evaluation tools, and videos, produced through the Hartford Foundation Initiative on GITT. Website: www.gitt.org

Administration on Aging International Website: www.aoa.dhhs.gov/international/SAGE-SW

Council on Social Work Education Website: www.cswe.org/sage-sw/

REFERENCE

Banozak, D. A., Mickus, M., Averill, M., & Clenda, C. C. (2000, October). Herding cats: Barriers to implementing a nurse aide educational program. *Annals of Long-Term Care, 8,* 10.

CHAPTER SEVENTEEN

Policies

WHAT IS A POLICY?

A policy is generally considered to be a written, guiding principle, directing work and procedures. Policies form the protocol for functioning, determine which personnel will be involved, and set up the delegation of responsibility. Social workers should be familiar with the nursing facility policies. In addition, they should know which policies designate their services.

WHAT AREAS DO POLICIES IN NURSING FACILITIES COVER?

There are two chief areas of policies in nursing facilities: facility personnel and residents. For example, a policy that would cover all personnel would be the Fire Evacuation Plan. A policy that would cover both residents and staff would be Resident Abuse, Neglect, and Mistreatment.

Policy formation is an important task. Some policies in the nursing facility are written to respond to government regulations, such as admission, transfer, and discharge policies. Other policies are written to provide the staff with a protocol of duty assignments for different situations that may occur in the facility, such as a resident threatening suicide. A policy for Resident Suicide would provide a staff intervention protocol including transfer and discharge to an acute care facility.

Policies reflecting government regulations are often key in the survey process. If the facility has a policy regarding, for example, resident grievances (the facility has the "policy" to provide all residents with an opportunity to have a grievance reviewed within 24 hours), it must adhere to this policy. Questions from state inspectors about resident/facility issues are often answered in the facility policy.

Some facilities have "policy committees"—staff members will meet on a monthly basis to discuss and review the existing policies and develop new policies, if needed. This committee can also be responsive to direction from the facility ethics committee if issues arise.

HOW DOES SOCIAL SERVICE CONTRIBUTE TO POLICIES IN A NURSING FACILITY?

Policies, particularly policies that relate to residents' rights advocacy or quality of life, should be regularly reviewed by the social worker. Social workers can help with the in-service education of the staff around specific policies, such as resident grievances or abuse. Other avenues of contribution are helping to revise older policies that pertain to the social service department or resident services, establishing protocols within policies and developing policies for issues that pertain to the care of residents in the facility. Social workers need to use their professional judgment around policy formation and contribute ideas and rationale that are pro-resident.

ARE THERE POLICIES FOR SOCIAL SERVICE DEPARTMENTS?

Yes. Most facilities have a policy manual that includes a detailed section on policies for the social service department. A typical policy section for social service would include: job descriptions for the employees in the department, any state mandated licenses, consulting, and specific descriptions of duties of the members of the department. These policies may or may not include responsibility for budgets, other advisory roles within the facility or corporation. Generally, there is an organizational chart to show the chain of command in the nursing facility and the position of the social service worker and department members.

Social workers should always review the policies for their departments at the time they are hired and make sure they are consistent with verbal agreements. Changes in staffing job descriptions, or title should be put into the policy manual as they occur. Routine reviewing of policies should occur approximately once a year and these reviews should be noted in the front of the manual.

PART FOUR

Surveys

CHAPTER EIGHTEEN

State Surveys and JCAHO Surveys

Both state laws and federal mandates require an annual survey of every nursing home that accepts Medicare and Medicaid payments. Surveys are conducted under the federal regulation umbrella and they have standardized formats. The dates of an upcoming survey are unknown to the facility. Facility resident care is reviewed by trained surveyors within the context of the areas of Administration, Nursing, Resident Rights, Kitchen/Food Services, and Environment.

Survey process utilizes a grid structure with points for each category. Problems with care or any other issues in the facility are addressed in survey within guidelines of what is called scope and severity and facilities receive a numerical score for each section. The maximum positive score a facility can receive is 132 points. The intent of this process is to encourage a more even quality of care in nursing facilities throughout the country (Massachusetts Department of Public Health, 2001).

WHAT IS MEANT BY "SCOPE AND SEVERITY"?

The scope and severity range matrix allows inspectors to categorize and score what they view in the onsite visit to the facility.

Scope is designates the number of residents involved. It is recognized that there are occasional situations in which mistakes are made. If an inspector sees a single instance of a facility employee making an error, this may be considered "isolated," such as failing to close a bathroom hallway door when a resident is using the toilet. On the other hand, for example, if the facility staff habitually fail to close privacy curtains while bathing or dressing all residents, this would be categorized as being "widespread."

The severity is the level of harm actually occurring to residents when the errors are made. This is a range between minimal harm and immediate jeopardy. For example, if all dining residents appear to have correct diets as ordered, except resident A who has a special diet order to reduce choking. Resident A is given resident B's tray and resident A chokes and aspirates. This isolated error could be considered an issue of actual harm.

Scope Range:

Isolated—when one or a very limited number of residents are affected and/or one or a very limited number of staff are involved, and/or the situation has occurred only occasionally or in a very limited number of locations.

Pattern—when more than a very limited number of residents are affected, and/or more than a very limited number of staff are involved, and/or the situation has occurred in several locations, and/or the same resident(s) has/have been affected by repeated occurrences of the same deficient practice. The effect of the deficient practice is not found to be pervasive throughout the facility.

Widespread—when the problems causing the deficiencies are pervasive in the facility and/or represent systemic failure that affected or has the potential to affect a large portion or all of the facility's residents.

Severity Range: Facility deficiencies are also graded on the severity of the problems:

Potential for minimal harm—Level 1 is a deficiency that has the potential for causing no more than a minor negative impact on resident(s).

Minimal harm or potential for actual harm—Level 2 is noncompliance that results in minimal physical mental and/or psychosocial discomfort to the resident and/or has the potential (not yet realized) to compromise the resident's ability to maintain and/or reach his highest practicable physical, mental and/or psychosocial well-being as defined by an accurate and comprehensive resident assessment, plan of care, and provision of services.

Actual harm—Level 3 is noncompliance that results in a negative outcome that has compromised the resident's ability to maintain and/or reach his highest practicable physical, mental, and psychosocial well-being, as defined by an accurate and comprehensive resident assessment, plan of care, and provision of services. This does not include a deficient practice that only has limited consequences for the resident and would be included in level 2 or in level 1.

Immediate Jeopardy—Level 4 is immediate jeopardy, a situation in which immediate corrective action is necessary because the facility's noncompliance with one or more requirements has caused, or is likely to cause serious injury, harm, impairment, or death to a resident receiving care in a facility.

WHO IS THE STATE SURVEY TEAM?

The state survey team, with authorization from Health Care Financing Administration (HCFA), is comprised of trained people usually including a registered nurse, social worker, and nutritionist, as well as other disciplines.

WHAT COMPRISES A STATE NURSING HOME SURVEY?

States are mandated by both federal and state laws to conduct on-site inspections of the facilities for compliance with state and federal laws. The focus is primarily on the regulations pertaining to OBRA. The state surveys occur every 9–15 months and they are unannounced, but most facilities have an idea of when they are "due" for survey. Reports are provided to the facility as well as posted publicly following the survey.

Here are some key headings that surveys focus upon (*Federal Register*, Part 483, Sub Part B, Requirements for Long Term Care Facilities):

- §483.5 Definitions;
- §483.10 Resident Rights;
- §483.12 Admission, Transfer, and Discharge Rights;
- §483.13 Resident Behavior and Facility Practices;
- §483.15 Quality of Life;
- §483.15(g) Social Services, (2, 3, i, ii);
- §483.20 Resident Assessment;
- §483.25 Quality of Care;
- §483.30 Nursing Services;
- §483.35 Dietary Services;
- §483.40 Physician Services;
- §483.45 Specialized Rehabilitative Services;
- §483.55 Dental Services;
- §483.60 Pharmacy Services;
- §483.65 Infection Control;
- §483.70 Physical Environment;
- §483.75 Administration.

In addition, there are over 150 regulatory standards that nursing homes must meet at all times. Many of these are interrelated.

WHAT DO STATE SURVEY INSPECTORS LOOK FOR?

States are federally mandated to provide inspections of the nursing facilities. The general focuses are resident nursing care, observation of resident rights, and the physical environment of the facility. Surveyors look, in particular, for good resident outcomes. Residents who are happy and voice few complaints generally represent a well-run facility. Whether it be end-stage issues, a resident who is dying, or a resident who is confused with Alzheimer's Disease, it is that individual's treatment and care that are of import. The actual resident care needs in the facility are evaluated, along, of course, with the written documentation.

Before coming to the facility, state surveyors review the previous years' surveys, a current report of the local ombudsman, and any other complaints or issues that may have come to the attention of the surveyors during the past year. All this information will have an impact on the types of issues the surveyors will be examining. If, for example, the facility was cited for physical restraints in the previous survey, the surveyors will closely examine the use of restraints in the current survey to ascertain whether the facility remains in compliance with its plan of correction.

The survey methods do not distinguish, in particular, what discipline covers a specific area. There are some designations, such as the mandate that facilities provide a social worker for nursing homes with beds over 120, but the survey system does not point out flaws within a particular discipline, per se.

Whenever a citation is made, the surveyor provides a specific example in the facility. The names are omitted, but the circumstances indicate the foundation for the deficiency citation and the level of severity. The following are a sample of deficiency citations (without specific examples) from several Massachusetts facilities in 1998–1999:

- Provide each resident who displays mental or psychosocial adjustment difficulty with appropriate treatment and services;
- Provide medically-related social service to help each resident attain his or her highest achievable level of well-being;
- Keep clinical records that meet professional standards;
- Provide social services for related medical problems to help each resident achieve the highest possible quality of life;
- Not use a resident's own money for items that Medicare or Medicaid pays for;
- Let residents refuse treatment or refuse to take part in an experiment;
- Provide care in a way that keeps or builds each resident's dignity and self-respect;
- Proper notice before transfer or discharge of resident;
- Resident's right to refuse certain transfers;
- Reasons for transfer or discharge of resident;
- Give the right treatment and services to residents who have mental or social problems adjusting.

Each of the above deficiency citations was graded in terms of the scope and severity of the problem and a description of the problem. Facilities also provided a date of correction. The scope and severity of the problems found were phrased in terms from isolated to widespread and potential for minimal harm to immediate jeopardy.

WHAT ARE QUALITY INDICATORS (QIS)?

Quality indicators (QIs) are based on the Minimum Data Set 2.0 and

cover the following domains, or broad areas of care: accidents, behavior/ emotional patterns, clinical management, cognitive patterns, elimination/ incontinence, infections control, nutrition/eating, physical functioning, psychotropic drug use, quality of life, skin care. These areas or domains do not represent every care category or situation that could occur in the long-term care setting, but they do represent common conditions and important aspects of care and life to residents. The QIs are also closely affiliated with the Resident Assessment Protocols (RAPs) a component of the Resident Assessment Instrument (RAI). (Zimmerman, 1999, pp. 15–16)

Areas of particular concern to social workers follow: Q13. Prevalence of behavioral symptoms affecting others, Q14. Prevalence of symptoms of depression, Q15. Prevalence of depression with no antidepressant therapy, Q16. Use of 9 or more different medications, Q17. Incidence of cognitive impairment. These components are risks outlined in the *Facility Guide for the Nursing Home Quality Indicators* (Zimmerman, 1999).

WHAT ARE THE SPECIFIC DESCRIPTIONS OF SCOPE AND SEVERITY MATRIX FOR CITATIONS?

The descriptions from HCFA are as follows:

Isolated/Potential for minimal harm—Least serious deficiency and is isolated to the fewest number of residents, staff, or occurrences. This deficiency has the potential for causing no more than a minor negative impact on the resident.

Pattern/Potential for minimal harm—Least serious deficiency but affects more than a limited number of resident, staff, or occurrences. This deficiency has the potential for causing no more than a minor negative impact on the resident, but is not found to be throughout this facility.

Widespread/Potential for minimal harm—Least serious deficiency but is found to be widespread throughout the facility and/or has the potential to affect a large portion or all the residents. This deficiency has the potential for causing no more than a minor negative impact on the resident.

Isolated/Minimal harm or potential for actual harm—This is a less serious (but not lowest level) deficiency and is isolated to the fewest number of residents, staff, or occurrences. This deficiency is one that results in minimal discomfort to the resident or has the potential (not yet realized) to negatively affect the resident's ability to achieve her highest functional status.

Pattern/Minimal harm or potential for actual harm—This is a less serious (but not lowest level) deficiency and affects more than a limited number of residents, staff, or occurrences. This deficiency is one that results in minimal discomfort to the resident or has the potential (not yet realized) to negatively affect the resident's ability to achieve her highest functional status. This deficiency was found to be throughout this facility.

Widespread/Minimal harm or potential for actual harm—This is a less serious (but not lowest level) deficiency but is found to be widespread throughout the facility and/or has the potential to affect a large portion or all of the residents. This deficiency is one that results in minimal discomfort to the resident or has the potential (not yet realized) to negatively affect the resident's ability to achieve her highest functional status.

Isolated/Actual harm—This is a more serious deficiency but is isolated to the fewest number of resident, staff, or occurrences. This deficiency results in a negative outcome that has negatively affected the resident's ability to achieve her highest functional status.

Pattern/Actual harm—This is a more serious deficiency and affects more than a limited number of residents, staff, or occurrences. This deficiency results in a negative outcome that has negatively affected the resident's ability to achieve her highest functional status. This deficiency was not found to be throughout this facility.

Widespread/Actual harm—This is a more serious deficiency but was found to be widespread throughout the facility and/or has the potential to affect a large portion or all the residents. This deficiency results in a negative outcome that has negatively affected the resident's ability to achieve her highest functional status.

Isolated/Immediate Jeopardy—This is the most serious deficiency although it is isolated to the fewest number of resident, staff, or occurrences. This deficiency is one which places the resident in immediate jeopardy as it has caused (or is likely to cause) serious injury, harm, impairment, or death to a resident receiving care in the facility. Immediate corrective action is necessary when this deficiency is identified.

Pattern/Immediate Jeopardy—This is the most serious deficiency and affects more than a limited number of residents, staff, or occurrences. This deficiency is one which places the resident in immediate jeopardy as it has caused (or is likely to cause) serious injury, harm, impairment, or death to a resident receiving care in the facility. Immediate corrective action is necessary when this deficiency is identified. This deficiency was not found to be throughout the facility.

Widespread/Immediate Jeopardy—This is the most serious deficiency and is found to be widespread throughout the facility and/or has the potential to affect a large portion or all the residents. This deficiency is one which places the resident in immediate jeopardy or has caused (or is likely to cause) serious injury, harm, impairment, or death to a resident receiving care in the facility. Immediate corrective action is necessary when this deficiency is identified (Massachusetts Department of Public Health, 2001).

WHAT IS THE SCORE THAT IS ATTACHED TO THE SEVERITY AND DEFICIENCY MATRIX?

The scoring for the results of the survey is based upon a point system which may vary according to the state's system. The scoring is based upon the grid, the points assigned for each grid, and a computation. This information and the resulting scores are sent to Health Care Financing Administration (HCFA).

WHAT HAPPENS WHEN THE FACILITY IS FOUND TO HAVE DEFICIENCIES, OR WHEN A PARTICULAR DEFICIENCY IS CITED?

Nursing facilities that have deficiencies must provide a plan of correction within a determined time frame, to correct the deficiencies. If there are severe deficiencies, or problems with the facility and corrections are not made in accordance with the plan of correction and agreed time frame, the facility can be subject to large monetary fines. The facility risks the loss of its Medicare and Medicaid certification. At times the facility admissions will be stopped, and ultimately the facility can be forcefully closed with residents being transferred to certified facilities.

It is not the intention of the state surveyors to close facilities. The primary concern of inspectors is to have the facilities give good care to residents in the nursing home. If the care is not found to be in accordance with federal and state guidelines, then surveyors will cite the facility in accordance with the state and federal laws in effect.

HOW CAN SOCIAL SERVICE DEPARTMENTS AVOID CITATIONS?

The social service worker is a member of a team. As a member of the team and an ancillary provider of service, and it is easy for the social worker to complete his work within a functioning, mutually supportive team.

If there are problems, however, with other components of the team, in particular, nursing, social service members may be cited as well. This occurs because the team provides resident care that overlaps in multiple disciplines. For example, if a unit nurse notes in the chart that a resident's spouse dies and fails to tell the social worker, the social worker cannot proceed with his role with the resident (e.g., working through the grieving process).

In order to avoid citations under these circumstances, the social worker must be assertive in the role of advocate for the resident. The social worker can improve communication by verbally providing assurances to the staff that his intervention(s) with the resident will be helpful, giving education/information around the particular topic or issue—either as an in-service or an informal discussion, and explaining the concrete advantages of mutual communication. Social workers who maintain regular visible presence on a unit, speak with staff regularly about residents, and follow up with staff requests around resident issues generally have good rapport and communication.

In summary, the social worker can

- document information in the chart carefully and thoroughly;
- help residents access their rights and choices;
- give in-services for staff members about residents' rights and choices;
- support good communication between team members;
- develop good care plans with information from the MDS, RAPs, and resident records; and
- participate in the evaluation and response to the quality indicators.

DOES THE SURVEY TEAM INTERVIEW THE SOCIAL WORKER?

The survey team may or may not include the social worker in the survey process. The social worker's relationship with residents and documentation may indicate a well-functioning provision of services to residents and families, and the survey team may focus in another area. On the other hand, if the survey team finds resident abuse or neglect, the surveyor may likely question the social worker about her role with these issues. Assuming they have followed accepted, ethical social work practice standards, social workers should not feel intimidated by surveyor's questions.

WHAT KINDS OF QUESTIONS DO SURVEYORS ASK RESIDENTS?

Surveyors, within the time limits of their visit to the facility, meet with the Resident's Council, and oftentimes speak with the President of the Resident's Council. They speak privately with other residents as selected, with families, and at times with staff members. These interviews are conducted in a private setting unless the interviewee requests a staff member present.

The focus of the surveyor's facility interviews is around the quality of life that residents are experiencing in the facility. *Survey Certification and Enforcement. The Long Term Care Survey Regulations, Forms, Procedures, Interpretive Guidelines* (1995) gave sample questions for surveyors to utilize in the inspection process:

Please tell me about your room.

Do you enjoy spending time in your room?

Is there enough light for you?

How do you find out about the activities that are going on?

In a group interview:

Have any of you or the group as a whole ever voiced a grievance in the facility?

How did staff react to this?

Did they resolve the problem?

Do you feel free to make complaints to staff? (pp. 5378–5379)

DO ALL THESE SURVEYS IMPROVE RESIDENT LIVES?

Yes. In fact, a fact sheet from the HCFA Press Office (1998, July 21) stated that there is "clear evidence of improvement, but problems persist."

There have been improvements with the reduction of antipsychotic medication since the implementation of the new regulations. However, there is an estimated 16% continued overuse of antipsychotic medication at the time of this report. Residents are also receiving more antidepressant medication, which is commensurate with the estimated nursing home prevalence of diagnoses of depression. There has been a decline in the use of indwelling catheters for nursing home residents, and an increase in residents who are utilizing hearing aids. Physical restraint use has decline from 38% to 15%. All of this has been helpful to the quality of life for residents.

WHAT PROBLEMS DOES HCFA SEE AS PERSISTENT?

The fact sheet (1998, July 21) from the HCFA Press Office indicated that the following were problems that have persisted through even the increased regulations and surveys:

- "Predictable surveys, allowing facilities to prepare;
- Not enough citations for substandard care, inadequate enforcement;
- Clinical problems of pressure sores, malnutrition and dehydration;
- Resident physical, verbal abuse, and neglect and misappropriation of resident's property."

WHO CAN YOU CONTACT FOR ASSISTANCE WITH STATE SURVEYS?

Each state has designated agencies to provide facility inspection and to service residents, families, and others with the opportunity to file complaints. The majority of states list surveyors under a department title of Aging or Public Health and/or Social Services. For example, in Washington, the long-term care surveyors fall under the Department of Aging and Adult Services Administration; in New York, surveyors are under the New York State Department of Health; in Massachusetts, surveyors are under the auspices of the Department of Public Health, Health Care Quality; and in Florida, the Agency for Health Care Administration administers surveys.

WHAT IS THE DIFFERENCE BETWEEN JCAHO SURVEYS AND STATE SURVEYS?

Primarily, the difference between the two surveys is that though the Joint Commission on Accreditation of Healthcare Organizations (JCAHO) has recently adopted more resident-centered foci, they are still heavily weighted toward structure and presence of policies and procedures, while HCFA has expanded emphasis on clinical outcomes and quality of life.

JCAHO accreditation is a separate entity, private, nonprofit, providing accreditation services to a majority of health care providers. Facilities pay a fee to have JCAHO accreditation. They do not pay a fee for state surveys. With respect to accountability, the public has no access to JCAHO's processes for setting and modifying standards; HCFA's processes are open to scrutiny through the practice of publishing proposed rules for public comment.

HOW DOES JCAHO ACCREDIT NURSING HOMES?

JCAHO accredits nursing facilities based on the results of surveys conducted on a triennial basis to assess compliance with JCAHO standards. Facilities are scored on the degree of compliance based on a five-point scale for each standard.

Score	Definition	Description
1	Substantial Compliance	The organization consistently meets all major provisions of the standard.
2	Significant Compliance	The organization meets most provisions of the standard.
3	Partial Compliance	The organization meets some provisions of the standard.
4	Minimal Compliance	The organization meets few provisions of the standard.
5	Noncompliance	The organization fails to meet the provisions of the standard.

Scores are aggregated, based on a series of algorithms, to scores in 35 substantive areas (called grid elements), grouped into 11 domains, such as resident rights, assessment of residents, improving performance, and so forth. The scores in these areas, in turn, aggregate to a single summary score for the facility.

There are five possible accreditation decisions based upon the scores a facility receives:

- Accreditation with Commendation,
- Accreditation,
- Accreditation with Type 1 Recommendations,
- Conditional accreditation, and
- Non-Accredited (Joint Commission on Accreditation of Health Care Organizations, 2001).

REFERENCES

Health Care Financing Administration Press Office. (1998, July 21). *Assuring the quality of nursing home care.* Washington, DC: Author.

Joint Commission on Accreditation of Healthcare Organizations. (2001). [On-line]. Available: http://www.jcaho.org/trkhco_frm.html

Massachusetts Extended Care Federation. (1995). Survey certification and enforcement. Dedham, Massachusetts.

Zimmerman, D. (1999). *Facility guide for the nursing home quality indicators: National data system.* Madison, WI: Center for Health Systems Research and Analysis, University of Wisconsin.

The Long-Term Care Ombudsman Program

WHAT IS THE LONG-TERM CARE OMBUDSMAN PROGRAM?

The Long-Term Care Ombudsman Program (LTCOP) began in 1972 for the purpose of advocating for the rights of residents in long-term care facilities and board and care homes. The program is provisioned under Title VII of the Older Americans Act, administered by the Administration on Aging (AoA), and is funded through the Department of Health and Human Services Administration on Aging. Utilizing both paid and voluntary staff the LTCOP was developed as community-based nursing home advocacy. The reason for this was primarily "Because the system throughout the United States is so terribly fragmented, and because each part of the system has its own priorities and agenda, the LTCOP frequently becomes the 'log jam breaker' in resolving complex situations" (Arcus, 1999, p. 202).

Every state, including the District of Columbia and Puerto Rico, has an Ombudsman Program. The program is also represented in "their statewide networks of almost 600 regional (local) programs" (National Long-Term Care Ombudsman Resource Center, 2000). This indigenousness component of the program allows for the flow of information, attention and advocacy to come from within the very community where both residents and ombudsman live. "In 1998, over 900 paid ombudsman and 7,000 volunteer ombudsman, working in 587 localities nationwide, investigated about 200,000 complaints made by 121,000 individuals and provided information on long term care to another 200,000 people. The most frequent complaints involved lack of resident care due to inadequate staffing" (Administration on Aging, 2000).

There is also a National Association of State Long-Term Care Ombudsman Programs (NASOP), and a National Association of Long-Term Care Ombudsman (NALLTCO). These organizations are very active in legislative activity to benefit the rights of older people in long-term care facilities.

WHO IS THE OMBUDSMAN IN NURSING FACILITY?

An ombudsman, basically defined, is a trained person who acts as a commissioner who investigates complaints, reports findings, and mediates fair settlements. In their larger mission, the ombudsmen are to seek better care through advocating within state and federal systems.

Depending upon the facility and the situation, the ombudsman can act as an immediate advocate for the residents, meet with staff, and/or attend meetings as a representative. Frequently, the ombudsman visits with individual residents and observes any obvious problems or issues that exist in the facility. The ombudsman can be considered an important resource for residents, and their families and friends. The ombudsman can explain how nursing homes are organized and regulated as well as inform residents of their rights. He or she is designated to assess nursing home strengths and weaknesses prior to state surveys. It is felt that only the ombudsman represents the resident, totally and uncompromisingly.

HOW DOES THE OMBUDSMAN WORK WITH THE NURSING FACILITY SOCIAL WORKER?

From the perspective of the social worker in a facility, the ombudsman can be a helpful resource in resolving difficulties with residents, families, or their friends. Indeed, if the resident and family member are agreeable, the ombudsman can be a member of a family meeting, a care plan meeting, or other facility meetings. In this role, while acting as an independent advocate for the resident, the ombudsman can potentially defuse explosive situations.

It is important to remember that both the ombudsman and the social worker are advocates of the residents in the facility. Both share the concerns for the welfare and rights of residents in the setting. As allies, the social worker and the ombudsman can be a powerful team, helping to better the lives of residents. The two can work as a team through dilemmas with mediation, compromise, and conflict resolution. It is important to remember that the administration, nursing staff, and other service providers also share advocacy for residents. Care is best performed for the resident, in a team format, whether the role is in housekeeping, laundry, or administration.

At the same time, residents problems and issues can be an area of stress. As with any highly charged situation, ombudsman, social workers and the facilities can be at odds with one another around the appropriate care and comfort of residents. It is necessary for the social worker to examine the role of each and determine the strategies to best help residents without resorting to territorial scrapping.

The social worker can assess the skills and expertise of the ombudsman in the facility and help to use this person to assist residents and their families. Ombudsmen come with a wide range of skills, interests, and backgrounds. Many, as volunteers, are retired professionals (nurses, physicians, and social workers) who have chosen this role as a meaningful part of their lives. Others are simply interested in helping elders and enjoy talking to the residents. Regardless of the background of the ombudsman, the role and the impact they can have on the lives of the residents is valuable.

HOW DOES THE OMBUDSMAN BECOME INVOLVED IN THE FACILITY?

The extent to which ombudsmen can become involved in a facility is somewhat varied. The formal mandate for the ombudsman, according to Title VII of the Older Americans Act is to provide the following:

- "identify, investigate and resolve complaints made by or on behalf of residents;
- provide information to residents about long term care services;
- represent the interests of residents before governmental agencies and seek administrative legal and other remedies to protect residents;
- analyze, comment on and recommend changes in laws and regulations pertaining to the health, safety, welfare and rights of residents;
- educate and inform consumers and the general public regarding issues and concerns related to long term care and facilitate public comment on laws, regulations, policies and actions;
- promote the development of citizen organizations to participate in the program;
- provide technical support for the development of resident and family councils to protect the well-being and rights of residents." (Administration on Aging, 2000)

Individual ombudsman may elect to provide the above named services to residents in a variety of ways such as individual visits with residents, meeting with families, and meeting with the staff in the nursing facility. Thus, the ombudsman's role can be seen as a blend of advocacy and mediation.

The involvement of the ombudsman with angry, hostile residents can be difficult in some settings because this can bring up adversarial situations with the facility administration. For example,

Miss King, a 74-year-old single woman, was frequently unhappy with her three roommates and felt the staff should give her preference around her requests. She frequently complained of being too warm in the winter and opened her window, frequently reducing the room temperature to chilliness. The staff was very annoyed with Miss King because they felt she was not considerate of her roommates, who were frequently cold after she opened the window. The administrator had become aware of the problem and had offered Miss King another room. She declined. The dilemma of the open window continued for the staff and Miss King. The facility ombudsman, having met with Miss King over several months, became an advocate for her. There were several subsequent meetings with the ombudsman, the social worker, and the administrator. The resolution of the problem evolved through negotiating a room change, offering a similar window view and a single roommate who also enjoyed cooler temperatures.

It is helpful for the social worker to meet with the ombudsman on a regular basis. Meeting regularly can provide the social worker an opportunity to develop a rapport with the ombudsman and find mutually agreeable solutions to resident problems. Confidentiality should always be observed when speaking with anyone about a facility resident. Though the ombudsman can, with permission of the resident or their legal representative, examine the clinical chart, this sharing of information does not extend to conversations about specific residents, unless of course, resident permission has been given.

HOW DOES THE FACILITY OMBUDSMAN PARTICIPATE IN THE SURVEY PROCESS?

The Ombudsman Program is a part of the state survey team review. Prior to surveying the facility, the survey team routinely requests the opinions and observations of the facility ombudsman. The facility ombudsman is considered to be a "frontline" observer of resident care and facility operation. Pertinent to the duties of nursing home ombudsmen is the focus on strong advocacy for the individual resident and overall resident rights.

The involvement of the ombudsman in the survey process can be seen as minimally non-threatening, at time helpful by the facility and/or surveying agency, or it can be fraught with tensions and hostility. The expectations of the ombudsman program as well as the individual facility ombudsman are extensive yet have varying implementation. The observations of the Real People Real Problems: An Evaluation of the Long-Term Care Ombudsman Programs of the Older Americans Act (1993) included these findings; "The ombudsman program activities of too many states are piecemeal, fragmented, and focused primarily on responding to complaints that relate to individual residents of nursing facilities. These states are not in compliance with the spirit of the program provisions as stated in the OAA; the offices of the state LTC Ombudsman programs do not function as a whole, statewide, unified, integrated program delivering a range of individual systemic, and educational efforts" (p. 3).

WHERE DOES THE LTCOP-COLLECTED INFORMATION GO?

There is a federal reporting process that includes all states with a LTCOP. The 1998 report, for example, included specific issues or categories of Access to Facilities, Enforcement, Staffing, Patient Care, Residents' Rights, and Ombudsman Program Issues. There is a breakdown of this information within the states and within the previously stated categories and subcategories. Overall, there were 163,540 complaints logged by the country's LTCOP in 1998. In the category of Quality of Life with subcategories of Activities, Social Services, Dietary, and Environment, there were a total of 30,992 complaints. Of these complaints in Fiscal Year (FY) 1998, 5,244 were in Activities and Social Services. Another subcategory, in the same FY 1998 report, indicated that there were 53,665 complaints about problems with Residents' Rights—28% being in the area of Abuse, Gross Neglect, Exploitation (Long Term Care Ombudsman Report—FY 1998).

WHAT ARE SOME OF THE CURRENT ISSUES OF ADVOCACY FOR STATE OMBUDSMEN?

Many ombudsmen have been concerned about the need for federal legislation around minimum staffing in long-term care facilities. Mark Miller of the State Long Term Care Ombudsmen for the Commonwealth of Virginia testified in a Senate Committee hearing,

> Inadequate staffing continues to be the single biggest barrier to providing residents with a higher quality of care. Ombudsmen across the country frequently hear about a single certified nursing assistant (CNA) having to care for 20, 30, or even 40 residents on a shift. This contributes to a higher risk of resident abuse and neglect including malnutrition, dehydration, and pressure ulcers. Quality care indicators, enhanced oversight by state survey agencies, and educational campaigns are all critical components to the quality care equation. But all these initiatives will fail to produce the desired result, if nursing homes do not have adequate numbers of well-trained staff. Inadequate staff equals inadequate care.

HOW DOES THIS IMPACT THE SOCIAL WORKER'S ROLE?

Social workers have always been engaged in advocacy roles, and their participation in the consumer-patient rights movement has blended well with the values of the profession. Added to this movement is Title VII under the OAA, which solidifies many advocacy related-functions. It is important that social workers know about the ombudsman program, especially the interrelated policy, program, and research issues (Netting et al., 1995, p. 355). Social workers, with positive ombudsman networking can utilize the ombudsman to enhance residents' rights in the facility and to help create better care for residents in the facility. In essence, the "ombudsmen are supposed to help identify and resolve problems on behalf of residents in order to improve their overall well-being. The ombudsman program works alongside other programs, groups, and individuals engaged also in efforts to improve the quality of care and quality of life of residents in LTC facilities" (National Academy of Sciences, 1995).

REFERENCES

Administration on Aging. Department of Health and Human Services. The Long-Term Care Ombudsman Report FY 1998 With Comparisons of National Data For FY 1996–98.

Administration on Aging. (2000). *The Long-Term Care Ombudsman Program.* [On-line]. Available: http://www.aoa.dhhs.gov/factsheets/ombudsman.html

Arcus, S. G. (1999). The long-term care ombudsman program: A social work perspective. *Journal of Gerontological Social Work, 31*(1/2), 195–211.

Miller, M. (2000) Testimony of the National Association of State Long Term Care Ombudsman Programs (NASOP) Available [On-line]. http://aging.senate.gov/fr10mm.htm

Netting, F. E., Huber, R., Paton, R. N., & Kautz, J. R., III. (1995, May). Elder rights
    and the long-term care ombudsman program. *Social Work, 40,* 351–357.
Real People Real Problems: An Evaluation of the Long-Term Care Ombudsman
    Programs of Older Americans Act (Summary). (last modified 3/15/00) [On-
    line]. National Academy of Sciences. http://www.nap.edu/readingroom/
    books/rprp/summary.html [2000, Dec. 27]

PART FIVE

Diagnoses and Treatment

CHAPTER TWENTY

Dementia

WHAT ARE "THE DEMENTIAS"?

The dementias are generally considered to be a cluster of neurological conditions that seriously affect the ability of a person to think, reason, and act independently. The primary area of loss for individuals suffering from dementia is memory. This loss can be mild or profoundly significant. Social workers should be sensitive to the impact memory loss has upon residents when they attempt to orient themselves to a new environment. "It seems plausible to speculate that if knowledge of our past is important to our sense of well-being in the present, it is also important for people with dementia whose hold on the past is becoming more ambiguous, hazy intermitted and transient" (Chapman & Marshall, 1993, p. 41). The following is a list of the most common disorders, Alzheimer's Disease, Vascular Dementia, Creutzfeldt-Jacob Disease, Lewy Body Disease and Parkinson's Disease. It is important to encourage residents and families to seek out a thoroughly identified differential diagnosis because of the variations in treatment that are available to residents. Social workers should be familiar with all the dementias, the physical and cognitive signs and symptoms as well as treatments available.

HOW DO WE DEFINE THESE DISEASES?

It is important for the social worker and staff to help families and residents understand that a diagnosis of a dementia is not a part of normal aging. Although there have been numerous studies about the hereditary connections between family members, a diagnosis of a dementia does not mean all subsequent family members will have the same disorder. Each person should seek independent assessments based upon her or his individual symptoms. How do we define these diseases?

Alzheimer's Disease has been labeled "the leading cause of dementia—a set of symptoms that includes loss of memory, judgment and reasoning, and changes in mood and behavior. Doctors describe Alzheimer's disease as a 'progressive, degenerative, irreversible dementia.' This is another way to say that the amount of damage done by the disease increases over time, the nerve cells in the brain degenerate or break down, damage does to the brain cells can't be repaired—there is no known cure for this disease" (Alzheimer's Society, 2000).

Creutzfeldt-Jacob Disease (CJD) "is a form of progressive dementia identified by abnormal brain cells that have a spongy appearance—numerous tiny holes where brain cells have died. CJD is a rare and fatal brain disorder." The disease is further described as including "rapid onset and decline. Early symptoms include lapses in memory, mood swings similar to depression, lack of interest and social withdrawal. The person may become unsteady on her feet. Later symptoms include blurred vision, sudden jerking movements and rigidity in the limbs" (Alzheimer's Society, 2000).

Vascular Dementia (VaD) or Multi-Infarct Dementia (MID) results from brain damage caused by multiple strokes (infarct) within the brain. Mild or severe symptoms can include disorientation, confusion and behavioral changes. "VaD usually has a sudden onset immediately following a stroke. Strokes may alter the person's ability to walk, cause weakness in an arm or leg, slurred speech or emotional outbursts. VaD may follow a stepwise progression, where function can deteriorate, stabilize for a time and then deteriorate again. The cognitive symptoms may vary, affecting some areas of the brain more or less than others (e.g., language, vision, or memory)" (Alzheimer's Society, 2000).

Normal Pressure Hydrocephalus (NPH). "The classic triad of dementia, gait disturbance, and urinary incontinence are diagnostic features of normal pressure hydrocephalus. Approximately one fourth of persons with a secondary dementia have NPH" (Carnevali & Patrick, 1993, p. 273). A rare disease, it is caused by an obstruction in the flow of spinal fluid. NPH may be related to a history of meningitis, encephalitis, or brain injury. This condition is often correctable with surgery.

Pick's Disease is a rare brain disease that, while closely resembling Alzheimer's in some ways, differs in certain key aspects:

- changes in personality
- blunted or excited mood and emotions
- loss of social restraints in the early stages of the disease
- less disorientation than in Alzheimer's Disease and intact memory
- "Its pathological process consists of narrowing of the frontal and temporal lobes, extreme shrinkage of localized cortical areas, and reduction in neurons in the affected areas. Senile plaques, neurofibrillay tangles, and granulovacuolar degeneration as seen with Alzheimer's Disease, are unusual with Pick's Disease" (Eliopoulous, 1993, p. 307).

Parkinson's Disease is a disease that affects the control of muscle activity, resulting in tremors, stiffness, and speech impediment. In the late stages, the disease can be present with dementia including Alzheimer's Disease. Drugs used in this disease can improve steadiness and control, but have no effect on mental deterioration.

Lewy Body Disease. Recognized only in recent years, this irreversible brain disease is associated with protein deposits called Lewy bodies. "The dementia associated with Lewy body disease affects: memory, language, ability to judge distances, the ability to carry out simple actions, the ability to reason. People with this form of dementia suffer hallucinations, for example seeing a person or pet on a bed or a chair when nothing is there. They may suffer from falls for no apparent reason, because their ability to judge distances and make movements and actions accurately is disrupted" (Alzheimer's Disease Society of Great Britain, 2000).

Two of the following core features are essential for a diagnosis of probably Diffuse Lewy Body Disease:

- fluctuating cognition with pronounced variations in attention and alertness;
- recurrent visual hallucinations that are typically well-formed and detailed;
- spontaneous motor features of parkinsonism (McKeith et al., 1996).

The social worker can assist with obtaining a clear history of the resident through a face to face interview at the time of admission. Through direct resident observation, asking family members and other significant people in the life the resident before admission, the social worker can assist in clarifying some of the symptoms presented in a diagnosis of Lewy Body Disease.

Huntington's Disease (HD) is a hereditary disorder characterized by irregular movements of the limbs and facial muscles. "HD is a devastating, degenerative brain disorder for which there is, at present, no effective treatment or cure. HD slowly diminishes the affected individual's ability to walk, think, talk and reason. Eventually, the person with HD becomes totally dependent upon others for his or her care. Huntington's Disease profoundly affects the lives of entire families; emotionally, socially and economically" (Huntington's Disease Society of America [HDSA], 2000). This disease generally has an onset in "mid-life, between the ages of 30 and 45" (HDSA, 2000) and this can mean admission to a nursing home may arrive at a much younger age for those with this disease. Ultimately this can be significant issue for younger families. Social workers can be very challenged by these younger residents because they often have younger children, the families are isolated from others in the facility because of the typical advanced age of other residents and the progressive nature of the disease. It is important for social workers to increase their knowledge of the disease, provide regular support to the resident and family members.

Depression. The National Institute on Aging has targeted common signs of Depression for older people and these are slightly different from the DMS IV's description. Older people have difficulties with chronic illnesses, deaths of loved ones, and changes in their work life that require adjustments. Therefore the following list is relevant if they symptoms last more than 2 weeks.

- An "empty" feeling, ongoing sadness, and anxiety.
- Tiredness, lack of energy.
- Loss of interest or pleasure in everyday activities, including sex.
- Sleep problems, including very early morning waking.
- Problems with eating and weight (gain or loss).
- A lot of crying.
- Aches and pains that won't go away.
- A hard time focusing, rementhering, or making decisions.
- Feeling that the future looks grim;feeling guilty, helpless, or worthless.
- Being irritable.
- Thoughts of death or suicide. (AgePage, 2001)

It is important for the social worker to assist with identifying depression symptoms in the elderly because; "Doctors are often treating older persons for several health problems and as a result may not recognize depression when it exists. Depression may sometimes be dismissed by the doctor as merely crankiness or moods of old age" (Cox, 1996, p. 132). Depression also can cause symptoms of memory loss, but when the disorder is treated the symptoms are reversible.

HOW DOES DELIRIUM RELATE TO DEMENTIA?

Delirium and dementia are at times confused. Delirium is a state that has an organic basis and more acute (sudden onset) than a dementia. There are a number of symptoms including "disturbed intellectual function; disorientation to time and place but usually not of identity; altered attention span; worsened memory; labile mood; meaningless chatter; poor judgment; and altered level of consciousness including hypervigilance, mild drowsiness, semicomatose status" (Eliopolulos, 1993).

The social worker's role as part of the team is to assist in the evaluation of the symptoms of the resident. A careful history of the symptoms, review and observation of the resident either in the pre-admission process or in the can help in differential diagnosis of either dementia or delirium.

HOW DOES THE SOCIAL WORKER
PROVIDE INTERVENTIONS?

The social worker can provide assistance and intervention for residents with diagnoses of dementia through

- assisting staff with an understanding of the disease(s) and the symptoms;
- providing the families with education, resources, and community referrals;
- providing the facility and staff with interventions to help with difficult behavior;
- advocating for residents;

- providing support groups for family members;
- encouraging resident and family interaction;
- encouraging the development of dementia-focused units where staff is specially trained to deal with these diseases.

REFERENCES

Age Page (2001). Depression: A serious but treatable illness. National Institute on Aging. [On-line]. Available: http://www.nih.gov/ma/health/agepages/depresti.htm

Alzheimer's Society. (2000). *Disease-related dementias home page*. [On-line]. Available: http://www.alzheimer.ca/alz/content/html/disease_en/disease-whatisit-eng.htm

Carnevali, D. L., & Patrick, M. (1993). *Nursing management for the elderly*. Philadelphia: J. B. Lippincott Company.

Chapman, A., & Marshall, M. (Eds.). (1993). *Dementia: New skills for social workers*. London: Jessica Kingsley Publishers.

Cox, H. (1996). *Later life: The realities of aging*. New Jersey: Prentice Hall.

Eliopolulos, C. (1993). *Caring for the elderly in diverse care settings*. New York: J. B. Lippincott Company.

Greenberg, J. S. (1995, May). The other side of caring: Adult children with mental illness as supports to their mothers in later life. *Social Work, 40*, 414–423.

Huntington's Disease Society of America. (2000). [On-line]. Available: http://www.hdsa.org/about/about.pl?what ishd

The Alzheimer's Disease Society of Great Britain. (2000). *Lewy body disease*. [On-line]. Available: http://easyweb.easynet.co.uk/vob/alzheimers/information/lewbody.htm

McKeith, I. G., McKeith, D., Glasko, K., Kosaka, E. K., Perry, D. W., Dickson, L. A., Hansen, D. P., Salmon, J., Jowe, S. S., Mirra, E. J., Byrne, G., Lennox, N. P., Quinn, J. A., Edwardson, G., Ince, C., Bergeron, A., Burns, B. L., Miller, S., Lovestone, D., Collerton, E. N. H., Jansen, C., Ballard, R. A. I., de Vos, G. K., Wilcock, D. M., Jellinger, K. A., & Perry, R. H. (1996). Consensus guidelines for the clinical and pathologic diagnosis of dementia with Lewy bodies (DLB); Report of the Consortium on DLB International Workshop. *Neurology, 47*, 1113–1124.

Mace, N. L., & Rabins, P. V. (1981). *The 36 hour day*. MD: The John Hopkins University Press.

SUGGESTED READINGS

Beaulieu, E. M., & Karpinski, J. A. (1981, November). Group treatment of elderly with ill spouses. *Social Casework, 62*, 551–558.

Greenberg (1995, May). The other side of caring: Adult children with mental illness as support to their mothers in later life. *Social Work, 40*, 414–423.

Mace, N. L., & Rabins, P. V. (1981). *The 36 hour day*. MD: The Johns Hopkins University Press.

Monaghan, D. J., & Hooker, K. (1995, May). Health of spouse caregivers of dementia patients: The role of personality and social support. *Social Work, 40*, 305–314.

CHAPTER TWENTY-ONE

Depression

HOW DOES A DIAGNOSIS OF DEPRESSION AFFECT THE NURSING HOME RESIDENT?

Depression and the diagnosis of Depressed Mood is an area that should be of significant concern to social workers in long-term care. Many symptoms that are presented by elderly clients, such as memory loss, weight loss, and confusion are significant for other physical ailments, but they are also manifestations of a depressed mood state. In addition, many residents enter the nursing facility with a secondary diagnosis of depression for which they are being treated with an antidepressant medication. It is important to determine if this diagnosis and treatment are recent. If the resident has had treatment for Major Depression for more than 10 years, an OBRA/PASARR screening is required before admission to the facility (See also chapter 8, Pre-admission and Admission). Social workers should be involved in the evaluation of the current treatment plans and goals for a resident's diagnosis of Depression and assist the team by observing for changes in the resident's presenting symptoms. (See also PASARR Pre-admission screening and annual resident review.) It is also important to determine if the current treatment has been effective for improving the symptoms.

WHAT IS THE ROLE OF THE SOCIAL WORKER WHEN THE RESIDENT HAS A DIAGNOSIS OF DEPRESSION?

During the admission to the nursing facility, the social worker should be involved in the evaluation process to determine whether there are any diagnoses falling under the OBRA/PASARR evaluation. A diagnosis or a medication can give a cue that a person is being treated for a mental disorder. Many elderly have been treated at home for a number of conditions that may or may not be listed upon admission to the nursing facility. Therefore a list of medications may indicate the presence of a mood disorder for which the person is being treated. The purpose of the OBRA/PASARR is to determine whether the prospective resident will be receiving adequate services in a nursing home.

Assessment has always been one of the most clearly defined aspects of social work. The expansion of social worker assessment to include screening measures for mental health risk among elderly people is consistent with social work practice goals and values. Case managers and social workers in health care settings, in particular, might consider including some form of self-report instrument as a part of routine geriatric assessment. There is ample documentation that the knowledge of positive test scores on depression screening tests increase the frequency with which physicians accurately diagnose depression in their patients (Dorfman, Lubben, Mayer-Oaks, Atchison, Schweitzer, Djong, & Matthias, 1995, p. 301).

The social worker should be familiar with the signs and symptoms of depression as well as the current modes of intervention, drug treatment, and psychotherapy. A resident may have had inpatient hospitalizations for depression in his past history. In the past it was not uncommon for inpatient hospital stays to also include electroconvulsive (ECT) treatments for depression. Social workers need to ask about how a resident recovered from any or all treatments for a mental disorder.

Talking to the resident, the family and others who have been involved with the treatment of the resident should help provide a baseline for the diagnosis and help identify what has been helpful in the past to remedy the depression, if this information is available. The social worker can also request an evaluation from the mental health team, the psychiatrist, or the psychologist to determine whether there are any other diagnoses present or provide additional treatment choices given the resident's mental health and medical condition.

Social workers also need to be sensitive and at the same time provide supportive treatment advocacy for the issues presented by the resident, who may not be forthcoming about a history of mental illness. Although mental illness and in particular treatment for depression do not carry the previous negative stigma, many people are still reluctant to be "labeled." There are also some family members who are resistant to acknowledging a resident's mental health treatment need. A resident's quality of life can be improved a great deal if she is properly treated for a diagnosis of depression. Social workers can provide education, support, reassurance, and access to residents and their families.

WHAT ARE SOME OF THE SIGNS AND SYMPTOMS OF DEPRESSION?

Social workers who work in nursing facilities have a variety of skills and expertise in the area of mental health. Only in those states where the license permits does the social worker have the authority to diagnose and treat a mental disorder. All members of the team, however, need to be aware of the signs and symptoms of depression and other mental disorders in order for an appropriate referral to be made.

There are a number of mood disturbances listed in the (DSM IV) Diagnostic and Statistical Manual IV, American Psychiatric Association (1994). One of the more common is the Major Depressive Episode. The DSM IV provides the criteria for the Major Depressive Episode as Five (or more) of the following symptoms have been present during the same 2-week period and represent a change from previous functioning; at least one of the symptoms is either (1) depressed mood or (2) loss of interest or pleasure.

(1) depressed mood most of the day, nearly every day, as indicated by either subjective report (e.g., feels sad or empty) or observation may be others (e.g. appears tearful)

(2) markedly diminished interest in or pleasure in all, or almost all activities most of the day, nearly every day (as indicated by either subjective account or observation made by others)

(3) significant weight loss when not dieting or weight gain (e.g., a change 0/more than 5% of body weight in a month), or decrease or increase in appetite nearly every day

(4) insomnia or hypersomnia nearly every day

(5) psychomotor agitation or retardation nearly every day (observable by others, not merely subjective feelings of restlessness or being slowed down)

(6) fatigue or loss of energy nearly every day

(7) feelings of worthlessness or excessive or inappropriate guilt (which may be delusional) nearly every clay (not merely self-reproach or guilt about being sick)

(8) diminished ability to think or concentrate, or indecisiveness, nearly every day (either by subjective account or as observed by others)

(9) recurrent thoughts of death (not just fear of dying), recurrent suicidal ideation without a specific plan, or a suicide attempt or a specific plan/ or committing suicide (p. 327).

The DSM IV also discusses the need for the professional to observe body language, and facial expressions that convey a "sad" countenance. At other times there may be psychomotor changes, that include agitation (e.g., the inability to sit still, pacing, hand wringing, or pulling or rubbing of the skin, clothing, or other objects).

It is important to note the DSM IV specifically stated that the major depressive episode "is not due to the direct physiological effects of a drug abuse, to the side effects of medications or treatments or to toxin exposure" (American Psychiatric Association, 2000, p. 327).

WHY HAS DEPRESSION BEEN UNDERDIAGNOSED IN THE NURSING HOME RESIDENT?

There are several reasons that would cause depression to be underdiagnosed:

- myths about older people and their mental status;
- chronic ailments where symptoms are similar;
- misuse of antipsychotic medications to treat similar symptoms;
- lack of skilled psychosocial expertise in facilities to make differential diagnoses; and
- prejudice around psychological "labels."

The use of hypnotic and antipsychotic medications was one of the areas of significant concern to the members of Congress around the passage of OBRA in 1987. Antipsychotic medication use has decreased from 33.65% before OBRA '87 to 16.05% after OBRA '87. This drop represents a 17.6% decrease/or all residents and a 52.3% decrease in residents on antipsychotic medications. Despite extensive professional dissemination of information regarding the serious side effects associated with these medications, and potential misuse and over use of antipsychotic medication in general, comparison of 1974 and 1976–1990 data (34.63% versus 33.65%) shows that there was little systemic change until after the implementation of OBRA '87 regulations. Antidepressant medication use increased from 12.64% before OBRA '87 to 24.90% after OBR4 '87. This rise represents a 12.3% increase for all residents and a 97.0% increase in residents on antidepressant medication (Kidder & Kalachnik, 2001).

The authors conclude that change, though there is an improvement in the use of psychopharmacologic medication misuse in nursing homes, The behaviors, habits, and attitudes that created the practices resulting in psychopharmacologic medication misuse were present in nursing homes for 30 years or more. This means that it will take more than the eight years that OBRA '87 regulations have been effect to change the practices of some individuals, particularly if these individuals work in facilities that choose to remain isolated from current knowledge and contemporary professional practice in geriatric psychopharmacology (Kidder & Kalachnik, 2001).

HOW IS DEPRESSION MONITORED IN THE NURSING FACILITY?

Depression is monitored in the facility by the care planning team (nurse, CNA, rehabilitation team, etc.). The social worker's rapport with the resident can offer both clinical support as well as observation for signs and symptoms of improvement or decline around the interventions. In addition, the attending physician may prescribe medications, the pharmacy consultant reviewer may evaluate the dosage of the medications, and there may be a mental health team involved. In some circumstances, the resident may be seen as an outpatient at a mental health clinic.

The nursing home team should address, in the resident's individual plan of care, any psychiatric diagnosis. Following the care plan goals and interventions, there should be quarterly review notes of improvement, stability, or decline by all disciplines.

In summary, the National Institute of Health (1991) has stated that depressive symptoms occur in 15% of community residents over the age of 65. It is important that this knowledge be carried into the arena of the nursing facility as well. In the nursing home the team provides a treatment plan for depression as they do with other resident diagnoses. Included in this plan are specific interventions to remediate the presenting, observed problems. As with other psychosocial issues, the social worker can provide key information about depression and help the other team members with identifying a resident in distress. Signs or symptoms of depression can be misconstrued as other problems and the social worker can assist team members in differentiating behavior representative of the disorder.

REFERENCES

American Psychiatric Association. (1994). *Diagnostic and statistical manual of mental disorders* (4th ed.). Washington, DC: Author.

Dorfman, R. A., Lubben, J. E., Mayer-Oakes, A., Atchison, K., Schwietzer, S. O., DeJong, F. J., & Matthias, R. E. (1995, May). Screening for depression among a well elderly population. *Social Work, 40,* 295–304.

Kidder, S. W., & Kalachnik, J. E. (2001). Regulation of Inappropriate Psychopharmacologic Medication Use in U.S. Nursing Homes from 1954 to 1997: Part II. [Online]. Available: http://www.mmhc.comlnhm/articles/NHM9902/kidder.html

National Institute of Health. (1991). Diagnosis and treatment of depression later life: Consensus statement. *National Institute of Health Consensus Development Conference, 9,* 1–27.

CHAPTER TWENTY-TWO

Antipsychotic Medication

WHAT IS ANTIPSYCHOTIC MEDICATION?

Antipsychotic medications are used to treat the diagnoses of psychosis and the severe behavioral problems seen in diseases causing dementia.

> In the elderly, the prevalence of various types of depression, anxiety, dementia, and psychotic disorders can be as high as 10% for the non-institutionalized persons and 50% for nursing home residents. For institutionalized patients, antipsychotics are the most prescribed drugs, yet special consideration is required when prescribing these drugs to elderly patients. (McManus, Arvantitis, & Kowalcyk, 1999, p. 292)

Antipsychotic medications have been targeted by residents' rights advocacy groups because of the high rate of use and negative side effects in the elderly. Eliopoulus (1990) notes, "Antipsychotics, also known as major tranquilizers, are started in small doses in the elderly and gradually increased if necessary. The longer half-life of these drugs in older adults makes the risk of adverse effects high" (p. 356). She further states,

> Elderly individuals often develop extrapyramidal effects while on antipsychotics; signs include drug induced parkinsonisms, motor restlessness, agitation, severe muscle contractions, dyskinesias, and tardive dyskinesia. Tardive dyskinesia, the most serious of these adverse effects, is displayed through rhythmic involuntary movements of the tongue, mouth, and face, head and neck jerking, and jerking or swaying of the body. Early detection of symptoms is important, since a dosage change or discontinuation of the drug can reverse these problems. Prolonged tardive dyskinesia is not reversible. (Eliopoulus, 1990, p. 356)

WHAT IS THE ROLE OF THE SOCIAL WORKER WITH REGARD TO ANTIPSYCHOTIC MEDICATION?

As a member of the facility team, the social worker should be familiar with the medications the resident is taking and the desired outcomes from the treatment regime. The social worker can observe behavior, talk with the resident, and help with the presentation of the treatment plan to the resident and the family.

Many facilities have a consent form for the resident/family to sign when an antipsychotic medication is prescribed. This is an important process of "informed consent." Social workers should advocate for residents and their families to participate as much as possible in the treatment process and expected results.

There may be times when the resident's prescription for antipsychotic medication changes. The social worker should be made aware of these changes by the nursing staff (perhaps in routine morning reports or in "rounds"). As a team member and observer of the resident's symptoms, the social worker can provide key information to the team and physician. For example,

> *Mrs. Jones, a 74-year-old married woman was admitted to the Willows Nursing Home for a diagnosis of a fractured hip and wrist. She presented as being a shy, somewhat reticent woman with significant dependence upon her husband. Mr. Jones, an elderly man of 78, had been caring for his wife at home and anticipated bringing her home subsequent to her recovery. About 2 weeks after her admission, Mrs. Jones began to exhibit symptoms of severe depression. Her husband observed these symptoms and told the nurses they should give his wife Stelazine. After several conversations with the resident, the physician and Mr. Jones, the social worker discovered the name of the psychiatrist who had been treating Mrs. Jones at home for a number of years. She was called and made a "house call" to the facility. She reviewed the case and re-prescribed the medication Stelazine for a diagnosis of psychotic depression. The psychiatrist explained multiple medications had been tried in the past, but Stelazine had been the most successful in treating her symptoms. After about a week of drug treatment, the resident's symptoms had not observably changed. In review of her symptoms, several of the nursing staff felt the medication was insufficient to treat the resident's problems. The social worker addressed the concerns of the staff in a follow-up discussion with the psychiatrist. It was reiterated that the medication would take from 4 to 6 weeks to take effect. Within 2 more weeks, her symptoms had improved and she was ultimately discharged to her home and the ongoing care of the psychiatrist.*

The federal survey process has considered antipsychotic medication to be a restraint and there are important factors to consider in some states when a resident has a guardian or needs a guardian. (See also chapter 25, Legal Representatives.) This information is important for the social worker to communicate to team members and families.

WHAT SECTIONS OF THE CHART INDICATE WHETHER A RESIDENT IS TAKING AN ANTIPSYCHOTIC MEDICATION?

The resident's chart contains the physician's orders and the diagnoses and medications prescribed are clearly outlined. Many printouts from the pharmacy that supplies the facility with medications will list a drug as being "antipsychotic" or "antianxiety" or "antidepressant." This list can also designate a use for the other medications being prescribed for the resident. This is a clearly indicated informational component next to the drug, taking the guesswork out of classifying the unfamiliar drug name. There should always be a corresponding diagnosis for the use of a medication; e.g., bipolar disorder might have a treatment order for medication of lithium, etc. Lithium would not simply be on the list of medications without a corresponding diagnosis. It is important to remember, as well, that not all diagnoses will have medications. There are times when the diagnosis is managed quite appropriately without medications through behavioral therapy, redirection, or advancement of the disease process for which the original diagnosis was medicated, e.g., Alzheimer's Disease.

Social workers who are not familiar with a resident's prescription medications can also look up the name of the drug in the facility's copy of the *Physician's Desk Reference* (2001) or in a more user-friendly book such as the Complete Guide to Prescription and Nonprescription Drugs by H. Winter Griffith (1996). In addition, social workers can access some information from such web sites as http://www.pdr.net.

WHEN DO YOU SEE ANTIPSYCHOTIC MEDICATION BEING USED IN THE NURSING FACILITY?

"The era of modern psychopharmacology began in France in the early 1950s somewhat by chance, with the synthesis of Chlorpromazine (Thorazine) as a potential antihistamine. Noted to have mildly sedating properties, Chlorpromazine was first used as a pre-anesthetic agent. Within a few years, it was found to be effective in treatment of psychotic symptoms" (Austrian, 1995, p. 240). As previously described, antipsychotic medication is used to reduce severe symptoms and behaviors associated with mental disorders. The closing of many psychiatric hospitals in the early 1970s, with the older residents being placed in nursing homes, familiarized staff with the benefits of these medications in treating the behavioral symptoms of older people. The result was that antipsychotic medication was freely utilized with all types of dementia and behavioral disorders, which unfortunately caused many residents to be overmedicated and subject to significant side effects.

The nursing facility team generally views specific symptoms such as biting, scratching, kicking, hitting, etc., as being problematic both for resident-to-resident interaction as well as for care issues. Nurses and certified nursing assistants use behavioral logs to track the number of episodes of this type of behavior and when it is observed. This finite shift charting on a behavioral log will allow for the summary of the particular behavior, when it most likely occurs, and how often. This record makes it easy to calculate the numbers of incidents at the end of the month. The team can look for the efficacy of non-medicinal interventions and may, if these are not effective, suggest a medicinal response.

When medication is begun, the continuous review of symptoms becomes very important to the overall care of the resident. If the number of episodes of agitated behavior are not lower than the number of incidents at the initiation of the medication, then there should be a reevaluation by the physician or psychiatrist (in some states a psychiatric nurse practitioner or physician's assistant may supervise medication changes). When there is evidence that the resident's symptoms are lessened, the protocol has been to reassess the dosage or type of medication. The treating health care professional may reduce the dosage, and reevaluates the resident's condition on this lower amount of medication.

WHAT ARE THE ADVERSE REACTIONS TO ANTIPSYCHOTIC DRUGS?

The point of reducing dosage of antipsychotic medications is to provide the least amount of medication with the most effective treatment of the symptoms. A resident who has an approved indication for use of these drugs, and who has had gradual dose reductions attempts—and the dose has been reduced to the lowest possible dose necessary to control symptoms—is clinically contraindicated for further dose reductions. The time frame for tapering medications is generally no more and possibly less than 6 months of therapy.

The social worker, as a part of the team, helps to monitor these medications and the behaviors of the resident. The observations of the resident can be through the social worker's notes, and/or the mental health clinician's notes. It is also important for the social worker to be sensitive to both the resident and the family's questions about antipsychotic medication. Families and residents can respond from opposite sides of the issue, "No, I never want that type of medication for my mother/father!" or "Why can't you give them something to quiet them down?" Knowledge of medications and the limits and benefits are helpful when talking with families.

WHO CAN HELP WITH QUESTIONS AROUND MEDICATION?

The social worker, as a team member, can ask other knowledgeable members about medications, such as the registered nurse, the attending physician, and the nurse practitioner. These professionals can contribute to the social worker's knowledge of the prescribed medications. In addition, the nursing facility generally has a pharmacy reviewer who looks at the charts and the medication residents are taking. This pharmacist is an invaluable resource for information about the antipsychotic medications as well as other medicines.

Social workers may also attend conferences and seminars where medications are discussed. For example, a new drug, such as Quetiapine, may be introduced to treat psychotic symptoms. Drug companies frequently present opportunities for health care professionals to participate in informational sessions about the products. By attending these conferences social workers in health care can obtain clearer information about medications. Although medication is not under the direct auspices of the nursing facility social worker, the information, response of the resident, and the ancillary resident needs relating to it, indicate that this subject is important for the social worker to know about.

REFERENCES

Austrian, S. (1995). *Mental disorders, medications, and clinical social work*. New York: Columbia University Press.

Diagnostic and statistical manual of mental disorders. (1994). Washington, DC: American Psychiatric Association.

Eliopolulos, C. (1990). *Caring for the elderly in diverse care settings.* New York: J. B. Lippincott Co.

Griffith, H. W. (1996). *Complete guide to prescription and nonprescription drugs.* New York: The Berkley Publishing Group.

McManus, D. Q., Arvantitis, L. A., & Kowalcyk, B. B. (1999). Quetiapine, a novel antipsychotic: Experience in elderly patients with psychotic disorders. *Journal of Clinical Psychiatry, 60*(5), 292–298.

Physician's desk reference. (2001). New Jersey: Medical Economics Co.

CHAPTER TWENTY-THREE

Mental Health Consultants

WHAT IS THE ROLE OF THE MENTAL HEALTH TEAM IN THE NURSING FACILITY?

The role of the mental health consultant in the nursing facility is both broad and vital. The mental health team can consist of a psychiatrist (MD), a psychologist (PhD or PsyD), an MSW social worker, a psychiatric nurse, a nurse practitioner, and a Master's degree clinician in either mental health or family counseling. Team membership varies from consulting team to consulting team. Generally the psychiatrist reviews the medications for the team, but in some instances, a nurse practitioner completes this task and the psychiatrist visits less frequently. One team member is generally designated as the "opener" of a case. There may or may not be an ongoing component of one-to-one or group therapy within the team.

IS THERE ONLY ONE CONTRACTED MENTAL HEALTH TEAM IN A FACILITY?

Mental health providers generally have a contract with a particular facility and there is generally only one mental health provider per facility. Mental health contracts vary from facility to facility, but usually these agreements cover the process of providing the specific psychiatric/counseling services in the facility plus emergency care arrangements for residents in need of immediate psychiatric hospitalization.

HOW ARE REFERRALS MADE TO THE MENTAL HEALTH TEAM?

The mental health team generally makes visits to the facility at the request of the facility staff. Resident referrals (with orders and approval of the resident's attending physician) can be initiated in a variety of ways, through the social worker, through the nursing department, or with a team approach. The social worker should be involved in all referrals to the mental health team and provide a social service assessment of the resident *before* the referral is made to the mental health team.

WHAT KIND OF ASSESSMENT DOES THE SOCIAL SERVICE WORKER MAKE BEFORE THE REFERRAL TO THE MENTAL HEALTH CONSULTANT?

The social worker is the resident's first contact for mental health services. She is designated as a social service provider by the facility because of education, training, and specific assessment skills. In addition, the social worker, as a team member, has the greatest information about the resident in terms of the family involvement, psychosocial factors, and overall behavior. A social service assessment for mental health services should therefore include the following:

- An interview with the resident, observing any behaviors or presenting symptoms of the problems. At this point, the social worker can look at what base-line performance is for this resident. Questions to keep in mind, for example, include, "Is this a new problem or is there a history of increasing difficulties?" "What has been the history of social workers' contact with this resident and family?" "Can you observe any overt, visible behavioral symptoms, e.g., motor restlessness, facial grimaces?" "Is the resident able to verbally express the problem or issue?" "How does he or she express the problem?" "Does the resident present the 'story' in a coherent, understandable context?" "Is the social worker able to form a relationship with the resident *at this time*, to offer support and encouragement?" The social worker can bring this information into the context of the problem as well as generate any potential resolutions.
- An interview with the nursing staff regarding the problem presented. The staff who bring a problem forward may perceive the resident quite differently from each other. The social worker can ask, "Does the problem occur for all staff, all shifts?" "How long has the problem been occurring?" "Are there any new medical problems, medication changes, or care changes?" "What types of interventions have staff attempted with the resident?" The staff can also evaluate their own strengths in dealing with the resident and the problem, that is, what works best.
- A review of the medical chart and previous social service documentation. The social worker can also review nursing assistant behavioral logs, to determine the history of the problem(s), and any patterns of behavior. The chart can reveal past efforts of interventions for a resident's difficulties as well as new medical problems or treatments.
- An interview with other pertinent team members; the CNAs who directly work with the resident on a regular basis are an important resource. If other team members know the resident, such as the recreational therapist, activities director, the rehabilitation therapists, occupational therapist, physical therapist, or the rehabilitation aide, they can be sources of

additional information. Depending upon the facility, dietary personnel and housekeeping staff can offer additional components of a resident's behavior or problem.

- Speaking with family members. As with any other referral, particularly for a resident who has a designated responsible party, it is important to speak with the family members. The skills of the social worker in discussing the difficulties of the resident, the history of the problems, and the input of the family are very important. The family can be supportive for interventions, or resistant to them. Families can also offer new information about the resident that may not have been shared previously.
- An evaluation. The social worker gathers all information together to form her assessment, and evaluates the resources available in the facility—including, of course, her ability to provide the type of short-term interventions necessary to remediate the problem.

WHAT KINDS OF SERVICES DO THE MENTAL HEALTH TEAMS PROVIDE THE FACILITY RESIDENTS?

Most consulting mental health teams' services consist of a variation of the following:

- assessment of the resident to determine a mental illness diagnosis or confirm a pre-existing one;
- reviewing the treatment plan including all medications and other physical diagnoses that may be affecting mood or behavior;
- providing in the chart all documentation associated with a clinical diagnosis;
- providing individual psychotherapy and/or group psychotherapy;
- providing behavioral intervention programs;
- providing individual quarterly reviews for psychotropic medications when psychotherapy is not necessarily provided.

Mental health consultants can also vary in their direct role with the team. Often these consultants will provide, at no charge, a certain number of in-services to the staff on psychiatric disorders of the residents. Others will, if requested, meet with the team for care plan meetings, or meet with families or unit teams to discuss their clients. Frequently, there are behavioral issues that the staff finds particularly difficult to "care plan," redirect, or treat. The consulting mental health team provides a resource for these issues.

WHAT IMPORTANT FEATURES SHOULD THE MENTAL HEALTH TEAM OFFER THE NURSING FACILITY?

It is important to remember that the mental health team is an independent *service provider.*

- Residents who are referred must have physician orders in the chart to be seen, whether it is for diagnosis, medication review, therapy, or a one-time evaluation.
- residents/responsible parties will need to sign a permission form for the mental health team to see a resident. Private fee schedules for mental health team evaluation or treatment should be in the admission packet.
- All mental health teams treat at the request of the physician; recommendations are to the physician and need his or her approval for changes in treatment, medication, or in some cases, hospitalization.
- Care plans should be specific about the goals and treatment of the mental health team and this should be incorporated into the overall plan of care for the resident. It is not adequate to simply state, "Seen by mental health team, PRN."
- It is the responsibility of the nursing facility to monitor and assure the quality and consistency of the mental health consultant team members in their treatment of residents. It is standard practice for the facility to have in their records, with the contact for the mental health team, a copy of all team members' licenses.

The mental health team members will most likely provide some or all of the following as a part of their evaluation and interview with the resident:

- an initial assessment—combined information from the chart and their interview with the resident;
- a Mini-Mental Status Exam with score;
- AIMS testing and score;
- a complete DSM IV diagnosis and plan of care, and specific recommendations.

WHAT IS THE SOCIAL WORKER'S ONGOING ROLE WITH THE MENTAL HEALTH TEAM?

It is important that social workers read the updated mental health team reports on a routine basis as well as meet with team members who are providing residents with a service. These meetings should occur regularly. This helps provide for continuity of the team in their treatment of the resident and affords the social worker an opportunity to network with other professionals around the mental health care and treatment of the resident. Observations and suggestions of the mental health team can help formulate a better approach to resident care.

The social worker can also provide a liaison with the staff around recommendations. For example, if a resident is being seen by the mental health consultation team for behavioral problems and there are specific interventions the staff will need to follow, the social worker can provide additional support to the staff. The social worker can also suggest where behavioral plans need adjustment. For example,

Mr. Kenney, a very thin, 72-year-old man, with a diagnosis of Parkinson's Disease, frequently refused his medications regardless of the explanations of the nurses. His medication was important for controlling his tremors, stiffness, and his overall quality of life. His noncompliance was often an issue of contention with the staff. The mental health counselor suggested a behavioral reward of a roast beef sandwich if he complied by taking his medication for a total week. Mr. Kenney agreed to this arrangement because he enjoyed the roast beef sandwiches, but he quickly returned to his patterned refusal of medication 2 days after the agreement was made. Observing the ongoing dilemma, the social worker, in a meeting with the mental health clinician, made the suggestion that Mr. Kenney needed a more immediate reward. Her recommendation was to use ice cream. The nurses would offer Mr. Kenney ice cream as a treat if he didn't refuse his medications. This system was very successful and Mr. Kenney's acceptance and compliance around taking his medications went up to 98%.

WHAT KIND OF FOLLOW-UP IS NECESSARY FOR THE FACILITY TEAM WORKING IN CONJUNCTION WITH THE MENTAL HEALTH TEAM?

Residents who are seen by the mental health team and for whom recommendations are made must have some related follow-up. In other words, if a resident has recently been diagnosed with depression and the mental health clinician is recommending an antidepressant medication, it is up to the facility to address this recommendation with the attending physician. If the attending physician does not wish to follow the recommendation, documentation of this decision must be made as well as an alternative facility response. There are times when the mental health clinician may wish to speak directly with the attending physician to support her recommendation or see if the physician may have a differing opinion and wishes to wait for clearer symptoms.

ARE THERE OTHER MENTAL HEALTH TEAM ACTIVITIES THAT WOULD INCLUDE THE SOCIAL WORKER?

While it is not the responsibility of the social worker to manage medication recommendations or deal directly with the physician, the plan of care for the resident with a psychiatric diagnosis is of particular interest to social workers:

- Assist the team in the evaluation for the need to be seen by the mental health team.
- Monitor for treatment and/or medication effectiveness.
- Monitor for side effects of medications.
- Monitor for changes when medication or treatment changes are made.
- Observe for behavior within the social environment.
- Assist the resident in accepting the treatment recommendations.
- Aid in the assistance or decrease of service as needed.

- Provide additional ancillary assistance as needed by the resident, team, or mental health clinician.

Social workers should also work with both the facility staff team and the mental health clinician or team to provide the most thorough treatment choices possible in keeping with the resident's choices and dignity. Residents have choices in treatment for mental health as well as other health care treatment in the facility. It is important for the social worker to maintain the resident advocacy role with regard to the treatment plan that the mental health service offers.

WHO PAYS FOR THE SERVICES OF A MENTAL HEALTH TEAM?

This is an important question. Medicare pays many providers. Others receive payment from HMOs (generally very limited), Medicaid, and the residents (private payment). This is an exceedingly important issue for the process of referral and one that needs to be shared with both the resident, responsible party, and the mental health provider. Social workers should assume only the responsibility of linking the mental health provider with the responsible party. It is the responsibility of the mental health provider to deal with payment arrangements.

WHAT IF SERVICES ARE NOT AVAILABLE BECAUSE THE FAMILY, RESIDENT, OR INSURANCE RESOURCE REFUSES TO PAY?

Mental health services can be viewed as any other service to the resident. If a resident refuses to have mental health services, this becomes an issue of self-determination and the resident clearly has this choice, unless it directly impacts their own safety or that of other residents.

A different issue arises if a resident's family refuses to pay for services. While a resident may have selected a responsible party, the needs of the resident may not always be appropriately met under this party's management. It would be important for the social worker and the facility team to carefully review the care needs of the resident. The social worker and the team can meet with the family to discuss care recommendations. Engaging the family member(s) in the caregiving process is an important step in helping the resident.

A resident who wishes to have mental health services that are not available because of an insurance payment issue presents a somewhat different dilemma. Some mental health providers are willing to accept the case on a sliding fee basis or for lower fees. At times, other arrangements can be made so that another provider may see the resident, where payment is not an issue. Social workers can advocate effectively for residents in these situations through discussing care needs with the staff and making direct contact with providers on behalf of the resident.

WHAT IS THE ROLE OF THE SOCIAL WORKER IN SELECTING A MENTAL HEALTH TEAM FOR A FACILITY?

The role of the social worker in obtaining a mental health provider is significant. As the primary person on the team involved with advocacy for the residents as well as the psychosocial issues of the residents, the social worker is in a pivotal position to examine the services of a mental health provider. Some of the questions he might ask potential mental health services are "What are the qualifications of the team members?" "Beyond the specific educational degrees of the mental health team members, what is their direct experience with residents in nursing facilities?" "Who will be offering the direct services to the residents in the facility?" "What is the philosophy of the mental health team with regard to residents' rights, care, and treatment; family issues, financial issues; and providing support to the staff?" "Are there any provisions for in-service training?" "What is the philosophy of the psychiatrist around medications?" "What is the follow-up agreement around prescribing medications?" "Does the mental health psychiatrist favor any particular medications over others?"

In summary, the social worker plays a crucial role in providing mental health support for residents, by reviewing their needs, making referrals, and providing follow-up mental health care for them. Social workers should remain actively involved in the psychosocial needs of the residents.

SUGGESTED READINGS

Aoke, N., Ishihara, M., Gujita, A., & Inagaki, H. (1990). Usefulness of DFDL scale to evaluate the functions of daily living of demented residents in nursing homes. *Clinical Gerontologist, 9,* 19–47.

Brink, T. L. (1979). *Geriatric psychotherapy.* New York: Human Sciences Press.

Lazarus, L. W. (1984). *Psychotherapy with the elderly.* Washington, DC: American Psychiatric Press, Inc.

Sloane, P. D., & Pickard, C. G. (1985). Custodial nursing home care: Setting realistic goals. *Journal of the American Geriatrics Society, 33,* 864–867.

CHAPTER TWENTY-FOUR

Groups in Nursing Facilities

WHY SHOULD A SOCIAL WORKER RUN A RESIDENT, FAMILY, OR STAFF SUPPORT GROUP IN A NURSING FACILITY?

Although social workers are extraordinarily busy with paper compliance and individual and family problems, attending often 3–7 meetings a week, the running of a group will afford the social worker an opportunity to provide services to a greater number of people. It will also help the social worker meet with a number of residents, families, or staff who would otherwise be met individually or perhaps not at all. Groups also help the social worker because when they are positively formulated, they can provide positive bonds and good social reinforcement for the members.

WHAT KINDS OF GROUPS ARE RUN IN NURSING FACILITIES?

There are a number of different kinds of groups that can be conducted in nursing facilities. Support groups, topic specific groups, self-help (e.g., "stroke" group, "men's" group), family support groups, and AA groups are just some of the groups that may occur in a nursing facility. Social groups are also fostered by Activities for programs and events. Groups occur, too, through the normal cycles of families and friends meeting at the facility. Meetings for care planning, family meetings, staff meetings, and committees can be defined as "groups" in the sense that they get together at a set time and place with others (secondary group) with a purpose or task. Sometimes institutional groups are organized to teach a specific task or develop social skills for residents or clients who are returning to the community.

WHAT ARE THE COMPETENCIES THAT ARE UTILIZED FOR GROUP WORK?

Morales and Shafor (1998) discussed three key competencies needed for group work whether the group is a treatment group or a team meeting:

1. *Knowledge of group structure and function.* The social worker needs knowledge of the phases of group development and skills in handling the power issues that characteristically arise in groups.

2. *Capacity to perform the staff role within a group.* They must be able to identify the criteria for selecting clients or others to participate in the groups, recruit and screen potential members, and conduct the initial planning activities (arrange time and place to meet, invite members) that allow the group to come together.

3. *Ability to engage in group therapy.* In therapeutic groups, a social worker is likely to be particularly active in guiding the group's process. The worker should have considerable knowledge about each member and lead the process to ensure that his goals for being in the group are met, while at the same time, the group's goals are being attained.

WHAT HAPPENS IN GROUPS THAT MAKE THEM IMPORTANT?

The group is the natural setting for socialization to take place. Friendships, cliques, or gangs are informally organized groups, but they help to provide a sense of belonging, structure the norms and values of a culture, and influence a person throughout his life.

Residents who are in a group form relationships that are similar to those they have had in the community. For example, if a resident is seated next to another resident in a sitting room and formally introduced by a staff member, you may observe the multiple social responses this evokes: a smile, perhaps a nod, a verbal greeting, at times a handshake, and then even a comment about the weather or a current news topic. This tiny gesture, an introduction, evokes all of these small nuances and draws the person out, encouraging socialization. A group builds upon these skills and helps keep and build new skills, despite mental, visual, and/or hearing handicaps.

HOW CAN THE SOCIAL WORKER IN A NURSING HOME START A GROUP?

Groups are important in nursing facilities and they are effective in reaching a number of residents, families, or staff at one time. Obviously there are slightly different processes and modifications for different groups, but there are some primary areas to consider before the social worker starts the group.

Schram and Mandell (1994) discuss ten key questions for establishing a group:

1. What positives and negatives should we anticipate before beginning to work together as a group? (This may be modified with less able participants.)
2. What phases or cycles is the group likely to pass through?
3. Why is this particular group needed? What is its central purpose? What are its secondary purposes?

4. What kinds of activities will help this group pursue its purposes?
5. Who should be included in this group? What kinds of people and how many?
6. What kinds of structures will help this group to do its work?
7. What will be the role of the designated leader? What other kinds of leadership roles will the group need?
8. In what kind of environment will this group flourish?
9. What kind of interaction will the members have with the leader and with each other?
10. In what ways can we keep checking on how well the group is doing? (p. 397)

WHAT KINDS OF GROUPS ARE MOST SUCCESSFUL IN NURSING FACILITIES?

All groups have the potential to be successful. One of the primary aids in helping a group to be successful in a nursing facility is to maintain a timely schedule while addressing the needs of the group, both in the sense of members' skills and their ability to tolerate extended interaction. Knowledge of the residents, family members, and staff members in the group can be very helpful to the social worker running the group.

As with many other issues, the success of a group depends upon the group members, the leadership, and the benefits the members derive from being in the group. For example,

Sherry Smith, a social worker at Advent Nursing Home began a group to support new family members. She had begun the group at the request of the administrator, who had felt the facility needed a "family support" group. Sherry developed informational flyers, discussed the group at a Family Council meeting, and telephoned individual family members to encourage them to attend the group. In addition, Sherry made the meeting times in the early evening to accommodate working family members. After 3 months and three meetings, the membership in the group of seven members had diminished to only two members and the social worker. Sherry decided the group, despite her efforts, was not going to be a success, and disbanded the group.

In a nearby town another facility offered a support group to family members as well. This facility had a designated Alzheimer's Unit. The social worker, Joyce Wayland, a new employee in the facility, had not begun the group, but had continued the long-standing support group for the family members of residents with Alzheimer's Disease. She generally had the meetings in the evening, served refreshments, and provided speakers upon occasion. There were four core family members in the group, which could range in size from 6–12 people every month.

In reviewing the two groups noted above what helped to make one group more successful than the other? Although both social workers were equally skilled, the family self-identification (i.e., "family member of a resident with Alzheimer's Disease") was not as clear for those in the Advent Nursing Home group. Other factors relate to the specific group members, the ability of the group members to interact comfortably with one another, shared goals, and personal agenda. Although the social worker's skills are important, these other factors can impact the success of any group.

WHAT KINDS OF STAFF GROUPS ARE IN NURSING FACILITIES?

One of the most helpful groups for nursing facilities is a staff support group. In some facilities, there is a bimonthly staff support group for certified nursing assistants and a separate support group for licensed staff led by the social worker or social work consultant. The groups offer an opportunity for the staff to share their concerns, explore new remedies, and give each other support and encouragement.

The topics in such groups can range from resident care issues, to families, to other staff. Serious problems are referred (if the group selects this option) to the administrator, who then in turn addresses them with the appropriate personnel. These groups are open-ended for membership and the members are regularly reminded of the confidentiality maintained in the group.

It is important for these groups to be offered in an atmosphere of positive acceptance and without suspicion on the part of the administration. In creating an environment of acceptance, the staff group can feel "heard" and begin to improve their interpersonal role with residents. For example,

Katie Issac, a social worker, co-led support groups for licensed nurses and certified nursing assistants. Both groups varied in their numbers from month to month, but generally there were 8–10 present at every meeting. When she and her consultant began the group, the director of nurses had been very supportive. When the director of nurses left, a new director who was less supportive and understanding to the groups replaced him. She felt the groups took valuable staff away from the units. The groups ceased for a couple of months and then the social workers advocated for the staff, reiterating the need to the new director of nurses. After some discussion and time negotiation, the groups began again.

At times, when there is a difficult situation with a resident or a family, there will be a request to develop a time-limited, task-focused group to deal with a particular behavior. Social workers in these small groups tend to provide the information and training to deal with sensitive matters.

REFERENCES

Morales, A. T., & Shafor, B. W. (1998). *Social work: A profession of many faces.* Boston: Allyn and Bacon.
Schram, B., & Mandell, B. R. (1994). *An introduction to human services: Policy and practice.* New York: MacMillan and Company.

SUGGESTED READINGS

Abramson, T. A., & Mendis, K. P. (1990). The organizational logistics of running dementia group in a skilled nursing facility. *Clinical Gerontologist, 9*, 111–123.

Agbayewa, M. O., Ong, A., & Wilden, B. (1990). Empowering long term care facility residents using a resident staff group approach. *Clinical Gerontologist, 9*, 191–203.

PART SIX

Legal Representatives for Residents

CHAPTER TWENTY-FIVE

Legal Representatives

WHAT AND WHO ARE THE LEGAL REPRESENTATIVES FOR HEALTH CARE?

In the event that a person cannot speak for himself, the legal system has devised categories of designates to represent the person under certain conditions. Although there are a number of ways a person can leave his preferences, the only current legal documents are

Power of Attorney (POA)
Durable Power of Attorney (DPOA)
Health Care Proxy (HCP)
Guardianship

Before the health care proxy (HCP) was created, living wills provided information about how the person would want to have his medical conditions treated. However, living wills generally required the services of an attorney and while some factors were covered, other types of medical conditions and treatments were often not addressed. As a result, the wishes of the person were not adequately protected. Living wills remain valid in some states and can form a basis of a person's intentions, they are not valid as legal documents in all states at this time.

DO COPIES OF DPOA, GUARDIANSHIP, OR HCP HAVE TO BE PLACED IN THE CHART?

Yes! The person must provide any and all legal authority when the resident is admitted to the facility or when these legal documents are obtained. In the absence of these documents, the facility must assume that they do not exist. Admission coordinators and social workers should assist in obtaining this important information. It is important to request follow-up information, if during the resident's stay advance directives and/or the designee changes. The quarterly care plan meeting is a good time to review any and all information pertinent to HCP, guardianship, and DPOA.

WHAT IS A POWER OF ATTORNEY?

A power of attorney is a document signed by the person (principal), providing someone else with the authority to take certain actions on behalf of the principal. These actions often regard monetary or financial issues, such as the writing of checks, payment of bills, sometimes the sale of property, and filing applications. Generally a power of attorney does not cover health care decisions and ceases to exist when the person is judged incompetent. Power of attorney is given while, and when, the person is legally competent, and can be revoked at any time.

WHAT IS A DURABLE POWER OF ATTORNEY?

A durable power of attorney often initially resembles a standard power of attorney. It almost always includes provisions for financial assistance. The durable power of attorney is generally noted as an addendum for health care. This is a special kind of power of attorney that provides for the appointment of another person to make health care decisions for the person if the person becomes unable to make decisions on her own behalf. The durable power of attorney for health care may be limited by the person in any way and be further limited in its authority by law. A durable power of attorney in most states can be executed by simply completing a form and having it witnessed. The desires of the person always preempt the powers given under the durable power of attorney for health care. The durable power of attorney is limited in its power and limited to the types of decisions that can be made on behalf of the person. The attorney-in-fact, acting under a durable power of attorney for health care is allowed to make decisions only when the principal (the person making the designation) is judged by the attending physician incompetent to make decisions.

UNDER WHAT CIRCUMSTANCES DOES A PERSON NEED A GUARDIAN?

Guardianships have been used to replace an individual's decision-making ability because the person (ward) is not able due to incompetence or incapacity. The determination of incapacity is determined by individual state statutes and often requires the statements of physicians and/or psychiatrists, psychologists, clinical social workers, and/or hospital records. Traditionally, people have sought guardianship for the following groups: the elderly, the developmentally disabled, the mentally ill, those with impairment from severe substance abuse problems, and traumatically brain injured. Veterans have also been included in guardianship petitions because of severe incapacitating physical injuries or mental disabilities associated with military service.

Individual states have statutes which describe the necessary proof and documentation to prove incapacity/incompetence and the need for court appointed guardianships. The level of incapacity for an individual can vary, even day by day, but generally, when guardianship is sought, the individual's ability to make decisions regarding health decisions and finances is in serious question.

The type of guardianship has changed substantially over the past few years to reflect the wide variation in a person's capacity to make what is seen as "competent choice." There are now greater rights for the individuals who are alleged to be incapacitated. In several states, including Pennsylvania, laws have passed to ensure the petitioned individuals have legal redress. For example, in Pennsylvania the following takes place when there is a petition for guardianship:

- Notice to the persons alleged to be incapacitated;
- Right to counsel for persons alleged to be incapacitated, and a requirement that the court appoint counsel for the alleged incapacitated person or a "guardian ad litem" in "appropriate cases;"
- Increased burden of proof and evidence required to prove incapacity; and
- Annual reports by guardians. (Evans, 1995)

WHAT IS A GUARDIAN AND CONSERVATOR?

All states create their own laws regarding guardianship, who will be a guardian or conservator, how the guardianship is created, and the extent to which these legal representatives have power over their charge. Many guardianship statutes started out granting plenary—total control of the ward: finances, health, admission to hospital, choice of surgery, residence, etc. All states have statutes that describe and define the nature and the responsibilities of guardians and conservators to the ward or individual.

Many states have adjusted the statutes and laws to reflect less plenary guardianships as the only solution to caring for individuals with impaired judgment. New Jersey, for example, has recently created a "Model Judgment" court process to determine the use of guardianship. This Model Judgment could involve the following:

> The probate court may require additional information that does not appear in the physicians' affidavits. For example, the court may request a functional or cognitive assessment by a psychiatrist or a psychologist, the care plan assessment from the long-term care facility in which the alleged incapacitated person residents, or an affidavit from a geriatric care manager regarding the individual's ability to make decisions in certain areas. (Whitenack, 2000, pp. 2–3)

Guardianship and conservatorship in Massachusetts fall under the jurisdiction of Probate Courts. The reasons for appointment of a guardian for any person is as follows: to protect the ward's person and property, to use the ward's property in the most efficient manner possible and to maintain proper care of the ward. In this case, the ward cannot enter into contracts, change residence, or consent for medical treatment. Only the guardian can provide consent.

The only exception to the guardian's power is when the ward is in a Massachusetts nursing home and receiving antipsychotic medication. In this situation, the guardian's authority for treatment is suspended, the ward falls under the need for a Roger's Guardianship, a court appoints an additional guardian who reviews the plan of care and consent for medication and treatment.

In other states, there is recognition that competence can vary. Some individuals are competent enough to make decisions about their day-to-day life activities and should be allowed to engage in this decision making. As a result, states have revised guardianships to reflect areas of independent decision making and the need for an alternate decision maker. For example, in New Jersey (Whitenack, 2000), guardianships have undergone revisions to reflect the concepts of "solutions that are the least restrictive and intrusive to a person's life and preserve the person's autonomy to the maximum extent possible while providing the necessary protections."

WHO CAN BE A GUARDIAN?

In general, guardians can be anyone over the age of 18 with a specific interest in the welfare of the individual, including but not limited to family, friends, and any agency within the executive offices of human services or educational affairs. The guardian may be an attorney who has worked with the individual over a long period, and who has a particular interest in his client. Attorneys also work with agencies, such as the Veteran's Administration, and family service organizations to provide guardianship services to specific clients.

Generally, if a person has a responsible family member and she is deemed incompetent, a family member is appointed. In the cases where there are not any family members available or the family members are in conflict, some states have court appointed agency guardians, such as Wisconsin and Florida.

The nursing facilities do not become the guardians for residents for two major reasons: (1) conflict of interests around financial responsibility and alternative decision making, and (2) the long-term responsibility of guardianship that would continue subsequent to a resident's possible future permanent discharge from the facility.

IS GUARDIANSHIP COSTLY?

Yes, guardianship can be costly. Filing for guardianship can range from $3,000–$4,000 depending upon the state and requirements of the petition. The time and the cost involved in becoming a legal guardian can be daunting. The petitioner must have, in the case of the mentally ill, a medical certificate at the time he petitions the court for guardianship appointment. The court may request of the petitioner that he be bonded, to protect the finances and property of the ward. The ward and all family members are notified and they may come to proceedings.

WHAT IS A TEMPORARY GUARDIANSHIP?

A temporary guardianship is an appointment in which a specific time limit is set. A guardianship that is temporary is frequently subsequently made permanent. Temporary guardianship ranges from 30–90 days in length.

It is important to note that the petitioner for guardianship needs to proceed and file to obtain full, permanent guardianship. Otherwise, the ward remains underrepresented. This issue frequently occurs when relatives or friends of a resident apply for temporary guardianship to help with the admission of the adjudicated, incompetent person into a nursing facility. Once this objective has been achieved, the family may fail to follow through with additional applications because the primary problem has been resolved. The difficulty with this response is that the resident has been declared incompetent and generally does not regain full "competency" in the generic sense, leaving her "incompetent" and without decision-making representation.

WHAT IS THE HEALTH CARE PROXY (HCP)?

The health care proxy is legal document under state law that enables the person to choose a health care agent to act on the person's behalf. The health care proxy becomes effective only when the patient's attending physician has determined *in writing* that the patient lacks capacity to make or communicate health care decisions. The patient can revoke the proxy at any time. Both Massachusetts and New York (see Sample Forms) have specific forms for designating a health care proxy. There is not a need for an attorney to fill out a health care proxy; however, there is a need for another person to witness the signatures of those involved.

HOW DOES THE HEALTH CARE PROXY DIFFER FROM THE LIVING WILL?

Living wills are also valid in many states. The primary difference is the living will can be very specific about care whereas the health care proxy is generally less specific, assuming the proxy will follow the express wishes of the individual. As these are individually state designated,

Some "living will" legislation applies only to terminally ill patients, not to patients who are incapacitated by illness or injury but may live for many years in severe pain, or to patients in a coma, or to patients in some other extremely disabled state. Therefore it may be advisable to draw up a durable power of attorney, which appoints another person to make decisions if someone becomes incapacitated. A number of states have enacted statutes expressly for decisions about health care, which provide for a simple form known as a medical durable power of attorney. (Papalia, Camp, & Feldman, 1996, p. 520)

As with living wills, some health care proxies are limited by the state law. It is important for facility staff to be familiar with each resident's living will or health care proxy, particularly if it is in effect. In Washington state, the stipulations for revoking a living will are

> You can change your Living Will (Health Care Directive) anytime if you are mentally capable. If you are not mentally capable, you can cancel your Living Will any time, but you cannot change what you have written or make a new one. You can cancel your Living Will (Health Care Directive) by:
>
> - Destroying it or having some else destroy it in your presence; or
> - Signing and dating a written statement that you are canceling the Living Will; or
> - Verbally telling your doctor, or instructing someone to tell your doctor, that you are canceling it. You, or someone you have instructed, must tell your attending doctor before the cancellation is effective. (Washington State Department of Social and Health Services, 2000)

Also, because states differ in their legal acceptance of an advance directive, it is important that the laws of the state in which the resident resides be followed. In Massachusetts, for instance, the living will is not a legally recognized document, unless it was made before the option of a health care proxy was available.

WHO CAN BE APPOINTED A PROXY?

Generally, under the state's laws, anyone who is 18 years old (the principal) can appoint anyone as their proxy. Exceptions to this rule are the administrator, operator, or employee of a health care facility such as a hospital or nursing home where the principal is a patient or a resident, unless that person is also related to the principal by blood, marriage, or adoption.

Health care proxies are not in effect until the physician deems the person unable to make health care decisions. This does not have to be a permanent condition per se. If a person regains her abilities to make health care decisions, then the designated person's appointment would cease.

WHAT ARE THE LIMITATIONS OF THE HEALTH CARE PROXY?

Essentially, once the person is determined by the physician to be unable to communicate medical decisions, the health care proxy designate is able to make any and all health care decisions that the principal could make, if this person were able. In addition, the designate has the right to speak with physicians, obtain all medical information pertinent to the decision-making process, including diagnosis, prognosis, and treatment of the illness or condition. The other limitations to the health care proxy are limitations that the principal has made, or a court order that specifically overrides the proxy.

WHAT ARE THE WAYS A HEALTH CARE PROXY CAN BE CANCELED OR REVOKED?

The health care proxy can be revoked for the following reasons:

- another health care proxy is signed later on;
- the principal legally separates from or divorces the spouse and the spouse is named as the agent;
- notification of the agent, physician, or other health care provider verbally or in writing, that the health care proxy is revoked;
- doing anything that clearly demonstrates a desire to revoke the proxy, for example, tearing up or destroying the proxy, crossing it out, telling other people it is void, etc.

Social workers should have a working knowledge of the legal choices and information for both residents and their family members. If residents or their families have further questions and are unclear as to their choices, an attorney specializing in elder law may be of some help.

WHAT IS THE ROLE OF THE SOCIAL WORKER?

Social workers should be aware of all legal representative options for residents in nursing homes. It is also helpful to provide residents and families the opportunity to discuss these issues in a value-free manner. Social workers can provide residents and family members with an Extended Values History Form that addresses the values and beliefs important to a person.

The social worker can assist family members with options and/or referrals in the particular situation presenting. Social workers can provide education to residents and their families: "1) definitions of terms and procedures, 2) changing, updating, and canceling care decisions, 3) specific elder care role expectations, 4) overview of legal and medical procedures, 5) forms and paperwork, 6) community and professional services" (Cochran, 1999, p. 60).

Social workers can also help provide information to the staff in the form of in-service training about the current available resources to residents as well as the right to make choices about their health care decisions. Based on their own backgrounds and experiences, staff can present varying views about end life decisions, advance directives, and resident choices. The social worker can help advocate and support resident decision making and help staff become more sensitive to resident choices when these may be in disagreement.

Ideally, the times to review the existing health care directives are at admission and at the annual Interdisciplinary Team Meetings. It is always important, however, to also review the advance directives when a person has had a change in family membership, or when health care needs increase due to an illness.

IF ADVANCE DIRECTIVES SUCH AS A HEALTH CARE PROXY ARE EASY TO COMPLETE, WHY DON'T MORE PEOPLE HAVE THEM?

There are multiple reasons why a person would not complete an advance directive. Neuman and Wate (1999) write:

> Consumers rate the rationale that their families know their treatment wishes higher than health care providers as a reason for failure to complete. This suggests that consumers may be over confidant with their family's understanding of authority, and willingness to carry out their wishes. Even with an advance directive, the integrity of the surrogate's decision is dependent on the quality of communication that has occurred between patient and surrogate as well as the surrogate's ability to suspend self interest to act for the patient. (p. 50)

Social workers can empower both the resident and the family members through discussions of resident wishes at the time of admission, or periodically through the care plan meeting times or during discussion of discharge.

In summary, the social worker's knowledge and expertise in the area of advance directives can play a significant role in advocacy. As many families and residents do not discuss these issues prior to placement, the role of the social worker to mitigate the discomfort and convey the permission to both the resident and the family to discuss these issues is of invaluable import.

REFERENCES

Cochran, D. (1999). Advance elder care decision-making: A model of family planning. *Journal of Gerontological Social Work, 32*(2), 53–64.
Evans, D. B. (1995). *Pennsylvania guardianship procedures.* [On-line]. Available: http://evans-legal.com/dan/guardian.html
Neuman, K., & Wade, L. (1999). Advanced directives: The experience of health care professionals across the continuum of care. *Social Work in Health Care, 28*(3), 39–54.
Papalia, D. E., Camp, C. J., & Feldman, R. D. (1996). *Adult development and aging.* New York: McGraw Hill Companies, Inc.
Rupp, S. (2001). Common questions: Guardianship. http://prairielaw.com/articles/article.asp?articleid=1392&channelId=28
Washington State Department of Social and Health Services. (2000). *Aging and Adult Services Administration. ASASA library.* [On-Line]. Available: http://www.aasa.dshs.wa.gov/Library/legalrights3.htm#lw
Whitenack, S. B. New Jersey supreme court approves "model judgment" for use in guardianship matters to encourage use of limited guardianships. [On-Line]. Available:

CHAPTER TWENTY-SIX

Finances in the Nursing Home

HOW ARE FINANCES RELATED TO THE ROLE OF SOCIAL WORK?

Although it may seem removed, finances in the nursing home become an important task of the social worker, particularly when residents do not have a family/responsible party and are unable to advocate for themselves. Social workers in cooperation with the facility business office, administrator, state and federal agencies can help with the coordination of residents' benefits rights, and assist with the resident obligation to pay for their care in the facility.

WHAT DO SOCIAL WORKERS NEED TO KNOW?

While social workers should be aware and knowledgeable about a wide range and variety of both federal and state financial systems (e.g., Social Security, Social Security Supplemental Income (SSI), Medicare, Medicaid, HMO benefit plans, etc.), this does not mean that they are obliged to fill out all Medicaid, Social Security, etc., application forms. Residents, their families, their guardians, and their responsible parties should be empowered by the social worker to assume their appropriate managerial control in this area. Social workers should be aware that payments made by Medicaid for nursing home residents do have some stipulations for cost recovery. This means, the state that manages the nursing home payments for a resident has the right to seek financial restitution from the resident's estate, if any, for the money spent. This includes individuals who are 55 years or older, when they receive Medicaid, and individuals in nursing facilities, intermediate care facilities for the mentally retarded or other medical institutions. States vary in the aggressiveness of recovery of spent funds, but since 1993 the federal government has required states to recover, from estates, the costs of Medicaid expenses.

There are limits on a state's right to recover Medicaid benefits. Recovery cannot be made:

- before the death of a surviving spouse;
- if the individual has a surviving child who is under age 21 or who is blind or permanently disabled; or
- against one's home on which the state places a lien, unless additional protections for siblings and adult children are satisfied (AARP research, 2000).

WHEN DOES A SOCIAL WORKER BECOME INVOLVED WITH FINANCES?

Social workers need to help and provide interventions for residents under the following circumstances:

- Residents who are unable to participate and who are without family members/responsible parties.
- Residents who have family members who are unable to participate due to their own infirmities.
- Residents who are at risk because they have uncooperative relatives.
- Residents who have been financially exploited.

HOW DOES THE SOCIAL WORKER INTERVENE?

Interventions of the social worker can range from acquiring a responsible party for a resident, such as a guardian or conservator, to filling out and filing applications so that the resident may financially access the care and services he needs. If the resident has been financially exploited, the social worker is mandated to report this situation to the Department of Elder Affairs. The resident can also have the assistance of an attorney through the local AAA if he requests this service.

WHAT ARE THE TYPES OF FINANCIAL SITUATIONS THAT MAY HAVE AN IMPACT UPON A RESIDENT'S STAY?

There may be problems with

- Health insurance coverage,
- Medicare,
- Medicaid (Title XIX),
- Veterans Administration payment,
- HMO coverage, or
- private pay status.

It is important for social workers to help both residents and families understand Medicare insurance that covers nursing home residents. For years, the standard application of benefits for Medicare subscribers has been, a hospital stay of 3-days can qualify the person for a skilled nursing home stay of a total of 100 days. Many residents and families *think* they will automatically be given the full 100 days of Medicare A coverage. They are often startled and unhappy when, as they see it, the nursing home rehabilitation team decides arbitrarily that the goals have been reached and terminates Medicare coverage well before the 100 days have passed. Although poverty has dropped for older people, in 1999, the median income of older persons was $19,079 for males and $10,943 for females. The major sources of income for older people was:

- Social Security (reported by 90 percent of older persons),
- Income from assets (reported by 62 percent),
- Public and private pensions (reported by 44 percent)
- Earnings (reported by 21 percent). (Administration on Aging, 2000)

With typical daily private nursing home costs between $95.00 per day and $250 per day, many elderly are in the position of having very limited income to pay for their care and must utilize savings/investments. This is often difficult for the resident and the family to accept because they often see needed nursing home care as part of an insurance package or as an entitlement. Emotions can also run high for family members who see their inheritances diminishing to pay nursing home costs.

WHAT IS THE SOCIAL WORK ROLE IN THESE CASES?

The social worker can mediate between the resident/family perception of benefit coverage and the facility view. When possible, the social worker should meet at the time of admission with the resident and family and candidly explain, perhaps for the second or third time, the typical scenario of Medicare qualifications and access of benefits. These types of meetings help to set the intellectual and emotional stage for the events that follow the nursing facility admission. During the resident's stay, reexamination of the goals and resident progress toward these goals should be outlined carefully, and included should be the financial payment for care. When Medicare benefits are concluded, in the opinion of the facility staff, both the resident and the family should be carefully advised of their rights to "demand Medicare billing" as well as the options around discharge from the facility and SNF unit.

WHAT IS MEDICAID (TITLE XIX)?

Medicaid (Title XIX) is a state operated program that is totally separate from Medicare. Doris Carnevali (1993) stated, "Medicaid is a program of funding to states in the form of grants from the federal government that provides between 50% to 83% of costs" (p. 75). The program covers both young and old indigent people who are impoverished and who qualify for coverage under state legislated laws. States individually set income and asset amounts and these can significantly vary from state to state. Currently in Massachusetts, for example, eligibility for this program in the nursing home is based on income and assets. Figures indicate that 80% of residents or more depend upon Medic-aid to pay for their stay in the nursing home. At this writing, eligibility limits for Medicaid (Mass Health in Massachusetts) are

- Income:
  $8,244.00 for an individual in the community
  $11,064.00 for a couple in the community
- Countable Assets:
  $2,000.00 per individual in the community or nursing facility

If a resident has a spouse, the asset limit is $81,960.00 for the community resident spouse and $2,000.00 for the nursing facility resident. If assets are jointly held, there is a 90-day grace period for the couple to separate their assets into two separate names/separate accounts. The social worker should encourage applicants to visit Medicaid offices to ascertain their benefits and needs. The information about program income, and asset levels at Medicaid offices is available to all applicants or social workers at no cost.

California offers Medicaid as well, Medi-Cal. Qualifications for Medi-Cal are currently

- Income:
  $7,200.00 for an individual in the community
  $11,208.00 for a couple in the community
- Countable Assets:
  $2000.00 per individual
  $3,000.00 per couple in the community (Cal-Med, 2000)

As with the Massachusetts example, California also recognizes the need for the spouse remaining in the home in the community to have a portion of the "liquid" assets. The limit, at this time, in California is $76,740.00 with $2,000.00 for the individual in the nursing facility. Frequently residents have incomes that are higher than Medicaid allows. This does not generally present a problem because the cost of nursing home care is so high.

There is often also a difference in income limitations between a person who is receiving Medicaid in the community and a person for whom Medicaid is paying a nursing home. There is often a higher cap or limitation on income for Medicaid eligibility for residents in a nursing home, however, even with substantial income, some residents are unable to pay privately for their care. Residents with this type of financial eligibility difficulty may be involved with spend-downs (where they pay the nursing facility and their medical bills privately for a time) then during the last month of a given year or period time, reapply for Medicaid.

WHAT IS AN ASSET?

Title XIX, Medicaid, considers assets to be anything of tangible worth that a person owns (ownership is determined through the designated social security number, for tax purposes). Families often have difficulty understanding that the money Mom saved over the years in the bank, that they have preserved by paying for homemaking services and medicines, is now considered an available resource to pay for her nursing home care. At the same time, there are many families who are savvy enough to have consulted an attorney well before the resident has needed nursing home care. Some have protected their family assets in legitimate, thoroughly legally, "tight" loopholes. This can result in the resident being eligible to receive Medicaid without touching the family assets.

Many states are very strict when it comes to transferring assets. There is the important warning of, "Do not transfer money or other valuable property without consulting a competent professional for advice. Medi-Cal will deny eligibility for an indefinite period of time to persons who apply for nursing home assistance within 36 months of giving away or selling resources for less than fair market value to anyone other than a spouse, or who make improper transfers while receiving Medi-Cal" (Medi-Cal, 2000).

WHAT HAPPENS WHEN FAMILIES TRANSFER MONEY OR OTHER ASSETS?

Residents or families who transfer money or funds from one person to another, or one account to another to acquire eligibility status for Medicaid are often those who are determined ineligible. (The exception to this rule is when there is a spouse in the community and the financial split occurs after eligibility has been determined.) Although Medicaid denial is a legal matter for the nursing home because of nonpayment for care, the social worker must protect the resident from inappropriate administrative discharge/transfer or treatment neglect while the payment matter is settled. It is naturally very frustrating for an LTC facility administrator to suddenly find herself the recipient of information that the resident who has been denied benefits under Medicaid because of the illegal transfer of assets is now staying in the facility for "free." This situation often takes place subsequent to previous form of payment, to the facility that has ceased, such as Medicare or VA contract.

WHAT IS THE ROLE OF THE SOCIAL WORKER IN THESE MATTERS?

Generally, it is the social worker who is asked to help sort through some of the dilemmas that surround the case. The social worker can initiate meetings between the facility administrator, the business office, and the family to help work out an appropriate plan of action around payment. Medicaid applications can be resubmitted with either more accurate information, or in some cases, indicating that the monies improperly transferred have been returned. Where families have already spent the money, Medicaid will often deduct the amount assumed available, and grant eligibility based upon this data. It would then be up to the nursing home's financial attorneys to reclaim the missing money.

The social worker, though an advocate of the resident, should not be put into the position of "bill collector." The tasks of the social worker are mediation, advocacy, and support for the resident. Residents who are experiencing financial troubles with or without the presence of family can be most distressed and fearful. At times these fears may be around inappropriate discharge, or for others the fear is not receiving the care they need. Whatever the case, the social worker can offer support and encouragement to the resident around receiving consistent services.

CAN THE FACILITY DISCHARGE THE RESIDENT FOR FAILURE TO PAY?

It is well within the rights of the nursing facility to issue a 30-day intent to discharge notice to the resident and family when payment is not forthcoming either through insurance or private pay status. In discharging a resident, however, the facility must assure the resident that the transfer and location will be safe and appropriate services are available. Facilities generally want to avoid negative publicity that may arise around a "forced" discharge, though they may well be in their legal rights to do so. Social workers need to advocate for the rights and the well-being of the resident, regardless of the financial snafus.

In the Long Term Care Ombudsman Report FY 1998 facility discharge was a highlighted issue. Some cited state examples:

(Indiana) IN—Many facilities do not make timely Medicaid applications or provide adequate assistance in accessing the Medicaid system, resulting in transfer/discharge for non-payment. Facility staff lack knowledge about the Medicaid system. Residents, family members, and legal representatives have no understanding of the system. (Georgia) GA—Some facilities fail to notify residents of their right to apply for Medicaid when their Medicare benefits are exhausted. Because the Medicaid reimbursement rate is lower than either the Medicare or private pay rate, facilities have little incentive to retain Medicaid eligible residents over those whose care will be reimbursed by Medicare, or those who can pay through private insurance or personal resources. (Tennessee) TN—Involuntary transfers and discharges, many of which are related to denied Medicaid, are among the most common problems faced by nursing home residents. Administrators do not want residents who have not been approved for Medicaid payment. (Long term care issues identified by state ombudsman, 1998)

Mediation between all parties is an important task in which social workers can engage to help the resident. In addition to meeting with all the various participants, from the facility to the government agencies, the social worker can help with concrete functions. Simplistic explanations of benefits at the outset help clarify coverage. The social worker helping to facilitate the application process by providing means to copy financial statements, helping to fill out the forms properly, and sometimes letter writing on behalf of families can help provide resolution. For example:

Mr. Wilbur Prentice, 92, had been at Dove's Nest Nursing Facility for 2 weeks when it appeared that his skilled services were ending. Mr. Prentice's physical condition was unstable, though not qualifying for skilled services. His physician, who had known him in the community, recommended that he remain in the nursing facility. A LTC screening form was completed with the anticipation that Mr. Prentice would apply for Medicaid. Mr. Prentice's daughter, Ms. Marie Cole, lived out of state and when she was notified of his status, she stated that she would take care of matters. Two months passed and the bill for Mr. Prentice's nursing home stay remained unpaid. The application for Medicaid was never filed. The business office, the nursing department, and social worker called the daughter's telephone number repeatedly without success. A third month passed, and though it appeared that the daughter visited on weekends, the bill for his care remained unpaid. The administrator decided to send a certified letter to the daughter and to the resident stating the plans of the facility to discharge him to his home in 30 days for nonpayment. The social worker felt Mr. Prentice's care would be compromised in the community, so she made final call to Ms. Cole. This last phone call was successful. The social worker explained that she was concerned about the problems and the potential for Mr. Prentice's discharge to the community. She also inquired about the welfare of Ms. Cole because she had not been answering her telephone. Ms. Cole responded by stating that she had been very ill and would pay the bill right away. Two days later she brought a check to the facility for the entire amount due. The social worker made a referral to the business office where arrangements were made to provide Mr. Prentice with substitute resources to help pay his bills.

The social worker in the above case was able to provide a positive conclusion to the situation through

- continued persistence in resolving the problem;
- concern for both the resident and the resident's daughter;
- follow-up interventions to ensure the problem would not be repeated in the future.

This case illustrates the need for all members of the team to work together to assist residents and resolve problems. The tensions around these problems can ignite into unfortunate decisions for residents, families, and administration. When the social worker utilizes skills of mediation, organization, and advocacy, the resolutions are favorable to all.

REFERENCES

AARP. (2000). AARP research: Questions and answers on Medicaid estate recovery for long term care under OBRA '93. [On-line]. Available: http://research.aarp.org/health/d16443_estate_1.html

California Registry. [On-line]. Available: http://www.calregistry.com/resources/medi-cal.htm

Carnevali, D. (1993). *Nursing management for the elderly.* Philadelphia: J. B. Lippincott Company.

Appendix A–D. Long term care issues identified by state ombudsman. (1998). *Long Term Care Ombudsman report FY 1998.* Administration on Aging, Department of Health & Human Services. Washington, DC 2000.

PART SEVEN

Ethics

CHAPTER TWENTY-SEVEN

Social Work Ethics

ARE THERE ETHICAL ISSUES IN LONG-TERM CARE FACILITIES?

The ethical issues in long-term care have become increasingly complex as regulatory agencies expand their involvement and our resident population becomes more frail. The implications and impact of OBRA (Omnibus Reconciliation Act of 1987), individual state regulations, Health Management Organizations (HMOs), and Medicare's new Prospective Payment Systems (PPS), upon the health care industry and nursing homes in particular, has raised new questions about how we provide and deliver health care to our elder population. Social workers, in particular, can be caught between regulations that appear to safeguard residents, but that often cause controversy in practical application. The realities of social work in the long-term care settings include our endeavors to provide the excellent, responsible care to our residents who are entitled to quality life, comply with increasing verification of actions and at the same time reflect the current system of medical care of both profit and nonprofit businesses.

HOW DO SOCIAL WORKERS BECOME INVOLVED IN ETHICAL ISSUES?

Social workers in nursing home settings, by the very nature of their role, are responsible for helping residents and their families through the bureaucratic labyrinth that now constitutes our health care system. Ethical dilemmas can occur during any component of contact with the social worker and the elder person and family member, from the pre-admission meeting through the discharge from the facility. Social workers in the nursing home are strongly aware of the stresses ethical issues constitute.

WHAT ARE AREAS OF SUPPORT FOR THE SOCIAL WORKER?

The social worker can use several sources for support around ethical issues:

- The NASW Code of Social Work Ethics.
- The Nursing Home Social Work Standards.
- Current books and articles about social work ethics.

The National Association of Social Workers' (NASW) expanded Code of Social Work Ethics (1996, pp. 6–7), covers "broad, sweeping areas of social work practice including service, social justice, dignity and worth of the person, importance of human relationships, integrity and competence." The Code further states: "A historic and defining feature of social work is the profession's focus on individual well-being in a social context and the well-being of society. Fundamental to social work is attention to the environmental forces that create, contribute to, and address problems in living." Charles Levy (1993) states: "On one hand, their (social organizations and agencies) ethics are a function of their relationship and responsibility to those they serve or represent; on the other hand, they are a function of their relationship and responsibility to their community and society" (p. 53).

HOW MIGHT PROFESSIONAL DISCRETION BE USED?

Charles Levy (1993) provided a body of questions to help the professional in the field address issues of importance. The social worker should utilize these questions in reviewing situations:

1. What principles of ethics are applicable in the practice situation, and to whom (or to what) are they applicable?
2. In relation to the social worker's primary responsibilities, how may priorities be justifiably ordered when ranking both the applicable principles of ethics and those (persons and interests) to whom they are applicable?
3. What are the risks and probable consequences to be taken into account by the social worker when making ethical judgments in a practice situation?
4. What considerations and values are sufficiently compelling to supersede the principles of ethics that might otherwise be suited to the practice situation?
5. What provisions and precautions will be required of the social worker in order to cope with the consequences of the social worker's ethical judgments and actions?
6. How can the contemplated decisions and actions be evaluated in the context of ethical and professional responsibility? (p. 53)

WHAT ABOUT TREATMENT CHOICES AND DO NOT RESUSCITATE (DNR) ORDERS?

Dilemmas of ethical consideration in nursing homes have long been associated with resident-to-physician treatment choices and nurse-to-resident treatment choices. Some of the key elements of debate have been "do not resuscitate" (DNR) orders, resident competency of judgment to select medical treatment, and assignment of substitute decision making when a resident lacks family members.

The social worker is particularly well positioned to assist both residents and families around these choices. Social workers can help by providing information to all parties, and developing and sustaining the rapport between family members so that decisions are made based upon the resident's wishes and past life's values.

Treatment choices, and specific issues, such as DNR, should be reflected in the policies of the facility. The social worker should be very familiar with the policies and assist both the staff and the residents and families around how these policies effect choices.

WHAT ARE THE ETHICAL ISSUES A SOCIAL WORKER FACES AROUND ADMISSIONS?

Social workers frequently fulfill a variety of roles in the nursing home. It is not uncommon for the social worker to hold the dual role as the admission coordinator as well as the provider of social services for the residents of the facility, particularly in smaller facilities. In many cases the social worker replaces the admissions coordinator in her absence. Although in the past, nursing home beds and subacute units were at a premium, there have been recent increases in the number of available nursing home beds and this has increased competition between facilities. The resulting phenomenon has been to stretch the variation of resident care needs from the extremely frail resident to the young person who has a psychiatric diagnosis. Stresses occur when nursing home management directives to the social worker are to obtain admissions with the highest Medicaid MMQ (Managed Minutes Quota) Scores or those with short-term rehabilitation potential, or those who have psychiatric diagnoses with which the facility as a whole is unprepared to cope. While social workers are aware of the fiscal nature of the nursing home and the need for income, they are also acutely aware of the resident-to-facility blend that offers the maximum care to those who live in the facility.

Ms. E., single, age 41, was admitted to Green Hills, a nursing facility entirely devoted to the care of frail geriatric residents. Her admitting diagnoses from the acute care hospital included an extensive inpatient psychiatric treatment history, a diagnosis of mental retardation, a history of alcohol abuse, fire setting, assault and battery upon her previous dormitory roommate, and kleptomania. Her lack of family support was significant. She had one sibling, a brother who was not in the local area and for whom the referral gave no phone number. His contact with her, noted on the referral, was very minimal. The history of the resident indicated she had been in multiple extended care settings and these placements had poor outcomes. She was presently waiting for a group home placement planned by her Department of Mental Retardation (DMR) caseworker. At admission, her payment source, Medicaid, Mass Health, was only approving her stay in the nursing home for 30 days.

The initial dilemmas for the social worker in this case included several areas:

- admission of a young person to a geriatric facility;
- admitting information describing a history of poor adjustment behavior;
- limited facility experience in providing care for young residents;
- potential issues of safety and security for other residents and the new resident;
- designing an appropriate plan of care to meet her needs;
- time-limited funding plan;
- a complex discharge plan coordinated by another agency without any family supports.

The first area was the concern for the prospective resident, Ms. E., and her need for a setting where she could receive the services and treatment for her multiple behavioral and emotional challenges. The second area of concern for the social worker was the safety and integrity of the other facility residents. A young ambulatory person, Ms. E., who had a history of assaults, could place other inadvertently agitated residents at risk for harm. These difficulties coupled with the payment resource, time-limited placement, could put this resident at risk for further poor discharges.

The social worker helped to manage this admission and pave the way for Ms. E. to have the supports and services she needed. Upon admission, the social worker spoke with the nursing staff on the unit and contacted the activities director to address some of the specific needs that this resident would have while in the facility. The social worker also immediately contacted the DMR caseworker and discussed the nursing home stay plan, the discharge plan, as well as the time constraints for the funding of Ms. E.'s stay. The DMR caseworker was concerned for his client. He agreed that the placement was a poor choice for more than a brief respite, because of the frail, elderly residents in the nursing home. He assured the social worker that the group home plan was "80% guaranteed."

This case did have a happy ending. The resident, much to the surprise of the facility staff, made a good adjustment to the facility and her roommate. She participated in the activity program and offered to help with other residents. She worked with her dedicated DMR caseworker who was very motivated to assist her transfer. When the caseworker took her to the group home, she expressed enthusiastic interest. After several visits at the group home, the plan for her move there was completed. Although there were several incidents of "sticky fingers" with other residents' possessions, the items were recovered by the staff and returned to the appropriate residents.

WHAT ARE THE ETHICAL ISSUES AROUND DISCHARGES?

Most facilities have designated the social worker as the "discharge coordinator." This is a natural role for the social worker as her knowledge of the team recommendations, community resources, and needs of the family have been shared during the nursing home stay. However, the realities of the nursing home industry are that admissions and discharges need to be coordinated with the facility census needs.

While discharges can be "on hold" they can also be encouraged because of different funding sources. The HMO, Medicare PPS, and Medicaid as well as the resident's own determination of how he will spend his own money contribute to the discharge process. In essence, discharges are not determined by only the presenting needs of the resident, the recommendations of the doctor, and the rehabilitation team.

Mr. M., a widower, 74, was admitted to Sunny Acres facility following a total left knee replacement. The HMO approved paid stay for 7 days. This was his second knee replacement; his right knee had been replaced 4 years earlier. Mr. M. had several other diagnoses including depression, anxiety, CHF, and insomnia. He was also addicted, by his own admission, to sleeping pills. He stated that the pills reduced his overall anxiety. While in the facility, his new attending physician had reduced his sleeping medication and this had infuriated Mr. M. As the days of his stay in the facility neared completion, Mr. M. became more and more anxious and expressed extreme fear of returning to his home. The HMO case manager was adamant in her refusal to authorize further pay for the nursing home care, stating that he could go to his daughter's home. Mr. M. refused to consider his daughter's home as an option, or to return as planned to his own apartment with services.

The social worker in this case worked with the HMO case manager, the VNA services, Mr. M., and his daughter around a third discharge option, to spend his recovery out of state with his elderly sister. Through a great deal of effort and negotiations, the HMO agreed to the service plan out of state. Although the discharge process in this case was extremely time consuming and awkward, the social worker felt that this plan benefited the resident and his needs. Unfortunately Mr. M.'s heightened anxiety around his discharge proved too much for his heart and he died of a cardiac arrest less than 24 hours before his planned discharge from the facility.

Mr. M.'s case illustrates difficulties encountered with managed care nursing home stays as well as the pre-admission plans presented to both the resident and the facility. The social worker needs to develop a resolution process.

This requires the placement of a high value on a particular ethical principle and may result in the deprivation of an additional interest of the resident. The ethical dilemma can be explained by both the utilitarian and denotological theories. The social worker may hope to arrive at the correct judgement which will promote the client's best interest and well-being. (Sasson, 2000, p. 15)

In our case example, though Mr. M. appeared to have progressed toward his goals in physical rehabilitation, his emotional status did not, and readiness for discharge even with home care assistance was *emotionally* untenable to him. His adjustment to the post-surgical pain in his knee had been difficult. His heightened anxiety, fears, and loneliness collided with the narrow evaluation of the HMO about his postoperative recovery. The social worker, in the attempts to respond to Mr.'s needs, remained focused on his wishes, and worked diligently to help him balance his physical needs, emotional goals, and fiscal situation.

DO NURSING FACILITIES HAVE ETHICS COMMITTEES?

Yes. Nursing facilities have been developing ethics committees to respond and address the increasing ethical questions that have emerged as the result of available advanced medical as well as end life choices. Ethics committees provide a forum for discussion of ethical and legal issues, provide staff education priorities, establish nursing home policies, minimize possible liability, and assist families of residents who are gravely ill.

Ethics committees can review both individual cases and provide retrospective reviews. Beauchamp and Childress (1994) discuss the Major Principles of Bioethics: 1. Respect for Autonomy, 2. The Principle of Nonmaleficence, 3. The Principle of Beneficence, 4. The Principle of Fidelity, and 5. The Principle of Justice. These components can be used to address the issues that come before the committee.

WHAT KINDS OF CASES DO ETHICS COMMITTEES HEAR?

The committee is generally used to review the decisions about dying and/or life-sustaining treatment, residents' rights, and competency. Committees can also be used to educate the facility staff, help develop policies, or serve as a forum for the airing and resolving of disagreements about clinical care.

The ethics committees are not empowered to make decisions around reporting or directing individual employees. The ethics committee consultation is generally charged with identifying a large component of a problem and possible resolutions. The following example is of an individual case brought before a nursing home ethics committee and illustrates the need for the committee to be thoughtfully responsive.

Mr. Kevin Roper, 55 years old, was admitted to the nursing facility, for a short-term stay, from a rehabilitation hospital for the continued treatment of severe burns to his legs and toes. He was a retired elementary school teacher who was living in elderly housing at the time. His injuries were sustained when he attempted to put out a fire in his kitchen wastebasket. He had a history of both drug and alcohol abuse.

The social worker and the patient accounts supervisor, referred this case to the Ethics Committee when it was learned that he had, with the help of a friend, hidden sums of money from Medicaid in another state. His apparent financial destitution had qualified him for Medicaid during the months previous to his admission to the facility.

The case came before the Ethics Committee because Mr. Roper's primary health insurance had ceased to pay for his stay and he was currently in the facility under a Medicaid contract. The issue was whether the information about his financial status should be shared with Medicaid authorities by the facility. The Ethics Committee discussed several points around this case:

- Clarification of his current need for care, e.g. diagnoses, prognosis;
- Clarification of his current payer, insurance, liability, other sources of payment;
- Clarification of his competency;
- Clarification of his relationship to the friend.

The Ethics Committee in this case was stymied by several points:

- The lack of clear, specific evidence about the suspected Medicaid fraud;
- The nature of the short-term stay of the resident, (he was to be discharged back to his home within 3 weeks of the review);
- The difficulties associated with payment for his facility stay if he should be removed from Medicaid;
- His need for continued nursing care and treatment;
- The competence of both the resident and his friend.

The Ethics Committee in this case did not make any recommendations to report. The committee did clarify, however, the issue of potential fraud with residents using the facility-generated applications and identified some points that the facility could further develop. While the decision of the Ethics Committee was not satisfying to the social worker, she was able to accept it. Mr. Roper progressed very well with his rehabilitation and he was actually discharge 2 weeks early to his previous apartment with community services arranged by the social worker.

WHO ARE THE MEMBERS OF A NURSING HOME ETHICS COMMITTEE?

Frequently the ethics committee members are representatives from all staff disciplines. An average committee may have a cross section of disciplines: attorneys, social workers, clergy, nurses, administrators, trustees (if any), nursing home administrators, psychologists, physicians, as well as lay people from the community. Under some circumstances, members of the community at large, a Family Council member, or Resident's Council member may be included.

The members of the committee address problems from the perspective of their discipline. It is important for all the members to identify with and try to gain a better understanding of their own personal values, as well as the values and code of ethics of their particular profession. As with other committees in the nursing facility it is important for all members of the ethics committee to respect the issues of confidentiality. Ethics committees should develop a protocol for the discussion and policies for the review of resident case material. Communication with one another, a sharing of interests, and a genuine concern for the residents will result in the committee becoming a vibrant, vital section of the facility.

REFERENCES

Beauchamp, T., & Childress, J. (1994). *Principles of biomedical ethics.* New York: Oxford University Press.

Levy, C. S. (1993). *Social work ethics on the line.* New York: Haworth Press.

National Association of Social Workers. (1996). *NASW code of social work ethics.* Washington, DC: Author.

Sasson, S. (2000). Beneficence versus respect for autonomy and ethical dilemma in social work practice. *Journal of Gerontological Social Work, 33*(1), 5–6.

CHAPTER TWENTY-EIGHT

Abuse, Neglect, and Mistreatment

WHAT IS THE NURSING FACILITY'S POLICY ON RESPONSIBILITY FOR ABUSE, NEGLECT, AND MISTREATMENT?

Abuse, neglect, and mistreatment are not necessarily common occurrences in long-term care facilities. All social workers, along with all other members of the nursing facility team, are generally considered mandated reporters. In all states, licensed social workers are to report suspected or actual abuse, neglect, or mistreatment. Reporting abuse does not mean that the social worker is liable for its occurrence nor true verification of its occurrence.

It is valuable for the social worker to be familiar with the definitions of abuse and carefully review the facility's policy on defining abuse, neglect, and mistreatment and their policy of the mandatory reporting law. Policies can vary significantly from facility to facility and the social worker should not assume that every facility, even in the same state or region, handles these issues in the same manner.

In most instances, facility policies designate one or two people to formally report an abuse, neglect, or mistreatment incident and information to the appropriate state agency. In addition, most facility policies specifically designate the social worker to be in the informational reporting "loop" so that the social worker can utilize this information to help resident adjustment. In other cases, the social worker is not a direct participant in the reporting process to the appropriate state agency, though he may identify the problem and initiate the process.

WHAT DEPARTMENTS OR AGENCIES DO STATES GENERALLY DESIGNATE FOR REPORTING ABUSE?

Generally there can be three departments that oversee elder abuse, neglect, and mistreatment in nursing facilities: Aging, Health, and Social Services. The facility should have the addresses and telephone numbers of these departments clearly posted in the facility and in large type. This information should be positioned in a place or manner that can be read by residents, families, visitors, and staff. Generally these agency names and telephone numbers are found posted in the front lobby of a facility or in a main hallway. In addition, some facilities post reporting numbers in staff dining rooms, and at various nursing stations throughout the nursing home. These state telephone numbers and addresses should be periodically checked for accuracy.

DOES THE NURSING FACILITY SOCIAL WORKER HAVE A SPECIFIC RESPONSIBILITY?

The social worker, as a team member is expected to be knowledgeable about abuse, neglect, or mistreatment. The social worker should be familiar with the definitions of abuse, neglect, and mistreatment and he should be able to identify problems that arise in the nursing facility. In addition, the social worker can be expected to help by participating in the resolution of the issue. For example,

A report of an incident (neglect and mistreatment) was made voluntarily by one facility to the Department of Public Health. The resident had one of her toes severed when a CNA had inadvertently closed a door on her foot. Neither the CNA nor the nurse on duty during the shift had attempted to address the matter any further than to treat the wound and place a bandage on the affected site of injury. Though the resident did not complain of pain because the injury sustained had been on her stroke-affected side, she was concerned about her ability to ambulate. She expressed these feelings to the social worker shortly after the incident, pointing to the bandage on her foot. In the days following the case, the situation received a great deal of attention through the facility's nursing department, the facility's legal department, and the angry family. The social worker continued to meet briefly with the resident over the next week and provided her support and time to talk about the incident. In addition, at the request of the administrator, the social worker also met with the family and attempted to reassure them that although the small toe was missing, the resident would be able to stand and walk, according to the physical therapist. The staff development coordinator provided in-service training and education around care and treatment to both the nursing assistant and the nurse.

In the case example, the resident was a victim of both neglect and mistreatment. Through the careless, neglectful handling of the resident, the nursing assistant caused the toe to be severed. The nurse, to whom the incident was reported, did not properly follow up and provide a more thorough medical intervention. This was mistreatment. Although everyone felt uncomfortable and guilty about the incident, the response of the team was less than adequate. The family and the resident were understandably angry and hostile.

The social worker was in the position to help both the resident and family. She worked with both the resident and the family to maximize the recovery process and reestablish faith in the facility's caregivers. The facility provided special follow-up for the nursing assistant and the nurse involved, but also included procedural information to other staff. The family was reassured and did not pursue discharge.

If a resident has been victimized through abuse, neglect, or mistreatment, the social worker should be available to assist with the recovery process for both the resident and family. Assistance can be through referral to a counseling service or agency, or direct casework by the facility social worker. All efforts should be made to reassure both the resident and the family that the abuse, neglect, or mistreatment will not be repeated.

THE FOLLOWING ARE GENERALLY ACCEPTED DEFINITIONS OF ABUSE, NEGLECT, AND MISTREATMENT

Abuse: There is usually a presumption that abuse has occurred whenever there has been some type of impermissible or unjustifiable physical contact with a resident that has resulted in injury or harm.

1. Physical contact with a resident may constitute abuse, if such contact causes physical or psychological harm to the resident.
2. Unjustified physical contact as long as it contributes to harm, even if it is not immediate, and indirect causes of harm may constitute abuse.
3. Physical contact with a resident for the purpose of retaliation against that resident is never justifiable and constitutes abuse.

Mistreatment: There is a presumption that mistreatment has occurred whenever medications, isolation techniques, or restraints are used in a manner that results in noticeable harm to the resident. This presumption is strengthened if the harm results from failure to observe accepted standards of medical nursing or professional practice. The question of whether mistreatment has actually occurred or not, will often depend on, 1. whether the action was for a punitive, rather than for a therapeutic purpose and/or, 2. whether the benefit of that particular medication, isolation technique, or restraint outweighs the risks of harm to the resident involved.

1. As in the case of abuse, there is no fixed rule on how much psychological harm is enough to warrant a finding of mistreatment; even minimal psychological harm may be enough.
2. In order to constitute mistreatment, during the use of the particular medication or isolation restraints that are in question, there must be an intentional, deliberate, or willful misuse resulting from carelessness or failure to observe accepted standards of medical, nursing, or professional practice.

Neglect: There is a presumption that neglect has occurred whenever a facility or individual fails to provide a treatment or service to a resident that is necessary to maintain that resident's health or safety, and that failure results in a noticeable deterioration of the resident's physical, mental, or emotional condition.

Actions or omissions resulting in deterioration of the resident's physical, mental, or emotional condition constitute neglect.

The following is a list of typically mandated reporters, though any individual can report suspected abuse, neglect, or mistreatment.

Audiologists
Certified Nursing Assistants
Chiropractors
Coroners
Dentists
Health Officers
Licensed Practical Nurses
Medical Examiners   .
Medical Interns
Occupational Therapists
Ombudsmen
Opticians
Optometrists
Orderlies
Pharmacists
Physical Therapists
Physicians
Podiatrists
Police Officers
Registered Nurses
Social Workers
Speech Pathologists

WHAT HAPPENS WHEN A COMPLAINT IS LOGGED WITH A STATE AGENCY?

Any time there is a complaint of abuse, neglect, or mistreatment of an elder a response from a state agency will occur. For example, in Washington state, there are

> Complaint Investigators—these staff are also qualified surveyors. Their primary task is to respond in a timely manner to public and facility generated complaints. An investigation of a complaint can take from one day to several days, and then a report is written for the complaint, if they wish to receive a report. If deficiencies are found, citations are written and the facility responds with a plan of correction. Because all survey staff are qualified surveyors, they can take part in the survey activity, or do complaints. (AASA Programs, 2000)

In some states, the results of the complaints are not provided to the person making the report.

HOW DOES PAST ABUSE, NEGLECT, OR MISTREATMENT AFFECT A PERSON'S STAY IN A NURSING FACILITY?

Our residents come from a variety of settings and family situations. Neglect, abuse, and mistreatment may also be a part of a resident's social history or create potential risk at discharge. The records from a referring hospital will indicate a "Protective Service" case when a resident has had a history of abuse or neglect in the community setting.

It is important when gathering social service information to ask both the resident and the family if there is a history of abuse, neglect, or mistreatment. In some cases, residents and their families may be reluctant to discuss the matter, and others may flatly deny that any problems existed in the community. Social workers should be aware of a self-neglect disorder that is called Diogenes syndrome, referring to the fourth-century Greek philosopher who reportedly admired lack of shame, outspokenness, and contempt for social organization (Quinn & Tomita, 1998, p. 57). This syndrome is not a medical diagnosis, but a cluster of behaviors and symptoms associated with significant social withdrawal, self-induced (and preferred) squalid living conditions and particularly poor hygiene. Excessive hoarding may also be a part of this syndrome. Residents with past histories of self-neglect and hoarding do not adjust well to institutional living and frequently do better with services in their own homes. In some cases, there may be some residual anger about the problems of the past and families or residents may accuse other family members of being the perpetrators or as being responsible. Regardless of the issue or response, it is important for the social worker to be aware of the potential for difficulties when a discharge back to the community is anticipated. In addition, it is important to protect the resident in the facility if a problem area is identified. For example,

Mr. H., an 83-year-old widower, was admitted to Green Lawns Nursing Facility for a brief stay, following a bout with pneumonia and exacerbated COPD. His son, Sonny, visited him and asked to speak with both the social worker and the nursing staff. He related that a niece, Candy, whom Mr. H. had raised, was quite volatile, unstable, and often harassed her uncle for money to resolve her personal financial problems. Sonny was most concerned that Candy would come to visit and upset his father as she had in the past. He did not want to have her barred from visiting and indeed there was not any legal basis for a restraining order. A plan to have any of Candy's visits monitored and held in a common room was an agreed-upon intervention with both the son and the resident. When Candy arrived to visit the facility on a weekend, however, the meeting was not well monitored. The staff had been very busy with other residents and families. Candy, as predicted, became angry with Mr. H., and was overheard to be screaming obscenities at him. Apparently, he had refused to provide her with the money she demanded. When the weekend staff intervened, Candy requested that a psychiatrist see her uncle, because "he was not normal." His discharge date was set for later in the week.

In this case, the social worker, after having been informed of the event over the weekend, met with the resident. Mr. H. stated that he had had a visit with Candy and she had been her usual self. Although there was concern about

Mr. H.'s return home and possible future badgering by Candy, it appeared that Mr. H. was resistant to take any formal steps against his niece. He was discharged to his home without further incident. In a follow-up phone conversation with Mr. H., it appeared that Candy had moved out of state. The follow-up home care plan had continued to offer him services and he was returning to his former active life.

HOW CAN THE SOCIAL WORKER ENSURE A SAFE DISCHARGE WHEN ABUSE IS SUSPECTED OR KNOWN?

There are some key points that the social worker must consider when looking at the abuse, neglect, and mistreatment issues and a discharge plan:

- ongoing physical safety for the resident;
- ongoing emotional comfort for the resident (e.g., freedom from threat of injury or abandonment);
- care needs to be met in a way that will monitor progress and encourage the resident to maximize his or her potential for recovery and independence;
- ongoing financial safety, and freedom from coercion and exploitation around money issues.

The social worker can begin a safe discharge process through having specific discharge meetings with the resident, family, and the team in the facility. Addressing the physical needs of the resident with the nurse, the rehabilitation team, or physical therapist can help to provide the concrete understanding of the needs of the resident. Supplying a specific resource to help when the person returns to the community further connects the person to a "lifeline" support to avoid isolation.

In situations where the resident and/or the family is resistant to meeting, and refuses participation, the social worker can assess the resident's competence for personal decision making. Presuming the resident is competent, the social worker can

- alert the attending physician as well as the community physician to the decision of the elder and the potential for an "at risk" situation;
- make a referral to appropriate community services for follow-up and provide a referral for specific necessary care in the home;
- make a referral to protective services for community follow-up.

The majority of discharges are not complicated nor are they fraught with multiple problems. As with any setting, however, the variety of residents and their family members provides us with a wide range of both problems and solutions for dysfunctional situations. Social workers should be objective, clear, and precise in their documentation of their actions in "troubled" discharges. As with other documentation, value judgments and subjective comments should be avoided. Careful recording of the observed problems and the solutions provided will be helpful if there are questions about the discharge plan at a later date.

WHAT ARE THE STATISTICS FOR ABUSE?

The prevalence of reported elder abuse in the general population according to Quinn and Tomita (1998) was 3.15% or 32 in 1,000 cases. The most common type of abuse was spousal abuse—wife to husband, 36.5%, followed by husband to wife, 22%—followed by son to parent, 16%, and daughter to parent, 8%. These authors further discussed abuse risks with "significant factors were alcohol consumption, and depression on the part of the caregiver, and socially disruptive behavior and communication problems on the part of the elder" (Quinn & Tomita, 1998, p. 34).

In a recent study in New York, Choi and Mayer (2000) addressed risk factors in elder abuse. One key issue they found was the financial exploitation:

> Like the self-neglect group, a majority of the financial exploitation group lived alone, while the majority of the physical/psychological abused and neglected lived with others—mostly family members. It is not surprising that the majority of perpetrators of physical/psychological abuse were spouses and adult children where as almost 40% of perpetrators of financial exploitation were unrelated to the victim. (p. 11)

Financial abuse and exploitation is most likely the least reported of the abuse cases. Embarrassment, unwillingness to prosecute the wrongdoer, confusion over the exploitation, and resignation around the loss are the chief reasons that elders underreport their experience. Financial abuse is also often difficult to prove, particularly if the elder is confused.

The National Coalition to Protect America's Elders is a watchdog group that has seen the situation of elder abuse and neglect in nursing homes unchanged from previous years. "The coalition pointed to a March 1999 General Accounting Office report that said one-fourth of all nursing homes in the country are not in compliance with federal and state regulations, despite the Health Care Financing Administration's possession of tools for enforcement" (Beaucar, 2000). These problems are tied into adequate, trained staff who provide the direct care of residents.

IN THE NURSING FACILITY, WHAT ARE THE RISK FACTORS FOR STAFF ABUSING RESIDENTS?

There are some key areas to alert nursing facility staff members to with regard to risk possible abuse.

1. *Staff members with a history of abusive relationships.* A history of abuse can have the effect of limiting the person's ability to solve problems effectively, primarily without resorting to verbal or physical attacks. Sometimes this can

translate into staff ineffectively dealing with a resident's resistance, or retaliating when behavior is viewed as being purposeful. Staff training can help provide a repertoire of alternative solutions to problems encountered by both certified nursing assistants and nurses.

2. *Holding high and rigid expectations of elder's abilities.* Elders in nursing facilities do not necessarily always improve through standard interventions. Their behavior may appear to reflect their intentions. The resident's actions, however, may not accurately indicate intent. It may be because of stroke or other neurological dysfunction. Staff may see residents who perform erratically with ADLs, or reject medications or treatment, as being manipulative or deliberately antagonistic. Helping to train staff to remain flexible, yet supportive to the care plan can assist in maximizing the quality of life.

3. *Holding high and rigid expectations of one's own abilities.* The amount of work in nursing facilities can be overwhelming; in particular, the expectations for paper compliance and the tremendous expectations of staff-to-resident ratio. For those who are determined to comply with every edict, the nursing facility setting can be excessively demanding. Helping staff to create reasonable personal boundaries and realistic self-expectations can reduce problems related to this issue.

4. *Difficulty discussing feelings with other adults.* The ability to share frustrations, to ask for help and discuss alternatives to the problems encountered daily is crucial. It is through talking and sharing, that the staff member can be more effective and less isolated.

5. *Using deceit or lies to "get the job done."* Staff is often under strict time constraints to achieve the end of a task for a resident. All residents are not completely compliant and staff may attempt to "short-circuit" the resident's resistance by lying, tricking, or otherwise deceiving. These techniques can erode the resident-staff relationship and ultimately create even more resistance through distrust. For example, residents can develop paranoid ideation around their food when food is used to mask medications they have refused to take in the past. Staff in-service training workshops can offer workable solutions, helping the staff member to develop honest, helpful alternatives to resistance.

6. *Frustration on the job or at home, when cooperation is not immediate.* Elders in nursing facilities are not always quick to cooperate. Some, if they feel pressure to rush, increase their resistance to caregiver urges, setting up conflict and controversy. Elders often seem to take a long time to respond to a request. When the demands are made in quick succession, residents can be overwhelmed by multiple requests. Staff can see the lack of response as resistance or stubbornness or deliberate malingering. In-service training can help this problem through role-playing and greater comprehension of the requests being made. Frequently residents attempt to cooperate, but their fledgling attempts are not always noticed.

7. *Difficulty or trouble controlling own temper.* Internal anger, rage, and impatience as responses to frustration lead to problems of controlling one's temper or an outward display of anger. In some settings, the need to respond quickly and with defensive meaning can be acceptable and even encouraged as a part of the "strong" image. Verbally snapping back at the offending person (resident or other staff member) is highly inappropriate and is labeled abuse. For exam-

ple, a staff member may feel entitled to respond to a resident's name-calling with a equal retort. Workshops, staff training, and adequate, available supervision helps to defuse these situations.

8. *Beliefs in the myths or stereotypes of elders.* The myths and stereotypes of elders can lead staff to ignore the resident as a viable participant in the care plan. Inadvertent abuse, neglect, or mistreatment can occur easily when resident requests and/or comments are assumed be irrelevant because elders are "forgetful" or "senile." Myths and stereotypes also interfere with helping residents to maintain their dignity.

In summary, the social worker can work with the staff to reduce some of these potential "hot points." Role modeling, education of staff through in-service training, and select problem-solving meetings can help reduce some of these stresses and bring into use more effective methods of dealing with resident behaviors.

REFERENCES

AASA Programs. (2000). Washington State Department of Social and Health Services. [On-line]. Available: http://www.aasa.dshs.wa.gov/Programs/FAQ.htm

Beaucar, K. (2000). Elder abuse is a crisis. *In the NEWS.* [On-line]. Available: http://www.naswpress.org/publications/news//0100/crisis.htm

Choi, N. J., & Mayer, J. (2000). Elder abuse, neglect, and exploitation: Risk factors and prevention strategies. *Journal of Gerontological Social Work, 33,* 5–25.

Quinn, M. J., & Tomita, S. K. (1998). *Elder abuse and neglect: Causes, diagnosis, and intervention strategies.* New York: Springer Publishing.

CHAPTER TWENTY-NINE

Confidentiality

HOW IS CONFIDENTIALITY DEFINED?

Essentially, confidentiality can be loosely defined as the element entered into when one confides, trusts, or is reliant. Confidence is also the state of feeling assurance, or reliance upon another person's secrecy and fidelity, as to tell in *confidence*. Some examples of confidentiality are: the attorney-client "privileged communication," the confessions heard by a priest, and the psychiatrist's/psychologist's client sessions, and more recently the social worker's client therapy sessions. Confidentiality extends to written records, taped sessions, private notes, and even appointment calendars. Courts and court cases have regularly requested records and do subpoena material. It is both the agency policy as well as the right of the client to withhold records or information based upon confidentiality and the obligation of the holder of records to uphold client privilege.

In the nursing home setting, residents and by association, their families are vulnerable in the area of confidential information held in the resident's medical chart. From the descriptions of the resident's previous life in the community, recorded on the Minimum Data Set (MDS), to the written or faxed referral from the hospital or home care agency, and the facts gathered by the interdisciplinary team at the time of admission, the chart is replete with personal data of varying depth. All of this information is to be held in confidence by nursing facility staff through ethical codes facility policies, state laws, and federal laws.

WHAT ARE THE EXCEPTIONS TO CONFIDENTIALITY?

There are general exceptions to confidentiality:

- Threats of suicide or homicide;
- Signed informed consents (e.g., releases indicating specific information to be shared with another party);
- Information shared during the resident's transfer or discharge to another facility or agency to ensure appropriate continuity of care;

- Abuse/neglect/mistreatment situations that require mandatory reporting.

WHAT DOES CONFIDENTIALITY COVER IN THE NURSING FACILITY?

The nursing home is bound by residents' rights to provide confidentiality of records for the resident's stay in the nursing facility. All charts containing information about the resident, the logs, or other material not in the medical chart can be considered private information as well (e.g., records pertaining to medications, treatments, or interaction between staff and residents). Confidentiality also pertains to records subsequent to the resident's discharge or death. Social workers need to be particularly vigilant in maintaining confidentiality around the disclosure of resident information to other agencies unless there is a written release. For example,

> Mrs. Wainwright was a resident at the Sunset Nursing Facility for 2 months. Her treatment, while a resident, included physical therapy for a fractured hip and ongoing treatment for her diagnosis of Depression with Melancholic Features. She had seen a psychiatrist in the facility twice, and was counseled by the facility social worker approximately twice a week. Her physical therapy was to be continued by the visiting nurses and her mental health care at home was to be continued by another psychiatrist. Mrs. Wainwright left the facility without providing the name of her community psychiatrist. A week after her discharge, the social worker received a call from a frazzled secretary requesting a faxed copy of Mrs. Wainwright's psychiatric care while in the nursing facility. The social worker declined to provide this without written authorization of Mrs. Wainwright.

The recent Health Insurance Portability and Accountability Act (HIPPA) of 1996 (December 2000) provides comprehensive federal protection for the privacy of health information. This regulation will be in full effect in 2002. HIPAA covers "All medical records and other individually identifiable health information held or disclosed by a covered entity in any form, whether communicated electronically, on paper, or orally in the final regulation."

The recent Health Insurance Portability and Accountability Act of 1996 (HIPAA) provided general national patient record privacy standards. In brief some of the areas covered are:

Consumer control over health information:
Under this final rule, patients have significant new rights to understand and control how their health information is used.

- Patient education on privacy protections. Providers and health plans are required to give patients a clear written explanation of how they can use, keep and disclose their health information.
- Ensuring patient access to their medical records. Patients must be able to see and get copies of their records, and request amendments. In addition, a history of most disclosures must be made accessible to patients.

- Receiving patient consent before information is released. Patient authorization to disclose information must meet specific requirements. Health care providers who see patients are required to obtain patient consent before sharing their information for treatment, payment, and health care operations purposes. In addition, specific patient consent must be sought and granted for non-routine uses and most non-health care purposes, such as releasing information to financial institutions determining mortgages and other loans or selling mailing lists to interested parties such as life insurers. Patients have the right to request restrictions on the uses and disclosures of their information.
- Ensuring that consent is not coerced. Providers and health plans generally cannot condition treatment on a patient's agreement to disclose health information for non-routine use.
- Providing recourse if privacy protections are violated. People have the right to complain to a covered provider or health plan, or to the Secretary, about violations of the provisions of this rule or the policies and procedures of the covered entity (Health and Human Services, 2000).

It is important for social workers to remember confidentiality when providing discharge services for the resident to other agencies, particularly in the use of FAX transmissions, or computer generated material. The referring material should exclude excessive material not necessary for the care of the resident. This would include any psychotherapy notes, which are held to a higher standard of protection.

ARE FAMILIES ENTITLED TO HAVE CONFIDENTIALITY IN THE NURSING FACILITY?

Yes, to the extent this is related to the resident. At times, some issues of the resident's family are brought into the facility. Sometimes these issues are brought up by staff familiar with a particular family because of the neighborhood of the facility and resident, at other times, it can be dysfunctional family issues spilling into the care setting. In any case, it is important to provide the families with courtesy and respect around sensitive topics. The NASW Code of Ethics also covers the issues of confidentiality for specific social work records.

HOW DOES CONFIDENTIALITY AFFECT A SOCIAL WORKER'S RELATIONSHIP WITH A RESIDENT IN A NURSING FACILITY?

Confidentiality has always been a part of the social worker's obligation with the client. In the case of the nursing facility resident, the social worker's role is circumspect within the facility setting and within the guidelines of facility policy, government regulations, and the state licensing board. A resident who requests that the social worker keep some piece information private, that is, not place it into the medical chart or share it with other staff, should feel comfortable that the social worker will comply. The only reason that the social worker could not comply with this request would be if the resident's care or safety was jeopardized. For example:

> *A resident states to the social worker that her son, in an angry rage, broke her arm 6 months ago. She requested that the social worker keep this information private for fear that she could not return home with him. The social worker explained to the resident that this information could not remain strictly confidential, because the resident's safety in the community was of great concern. The social worker supported the resident's desire to return to the community as well as to be safe. The resident was at first fearful her placement at the nursing facility would be permanent, but after reassurances that her community discharge plan was not jeopardized, she agreed to interventions of Protective Services and family counseling before and following discharge.*

The principle of confidentiality applies to the relationship between social worker and client. The social worker is also ethically responsible to tell the client the truth about those agency policies and procedures that will limit the extent to which she will be free to honor the principle of confidentiality. In addition, the social worker is ethically responsible to be clear and forthright about the manner in which treatment will be conducted, and the roles that both social worker and client will be playing. The social worker respects the client's right to self-determination in all matter affecting the client's life (Levy, 1993, p. 67).

ARE ANY PARTS OF THE CHART MORE CONFIDENTIAL THAN OTHERS?

Resident charts in nursing facilities are in the total sense, all confidential. Basically this means that from the dietitian's notes, to the CNAs record of bowel movements, to the psychiatrist's evaluation, the information is under the guidelines of confidentiality. The information should be treated with the same respect and privacy regardless of the "header" for the section.

WHO CAN HAVE ACCESS TO THE CHART?

Residents may read their own charts. Generally there is facility policy that dictates how this is presented and processed. In many settings, residents who request to read their charts are provided with a staff member to interpret the information. Some facilities have policies that request residents who wish to read their chart provide the facility with some advanced notification. Residents' family members, as well as the facility ombudsman, may read the resident charts, but this is only with permission of the resident or guardian.

State survey teams, or other governing or licensing bodies also have the right to review the chart and the contents. They are also bound by confidentiality not to divulge the information. Anyone who provides care for the resident is also allowed to review, and/or read all parts of the chart. For example, the physical therapist may read the nursing notes as well as the CNAs behavioral logs to determine the physical or emotional status of the resident he is treating. The consultant pharmacist will read the chart in order to determine his recommendations for medications. However, the maintenance supervisor, the building manager, or a physician who is not treating the resident cannot read the charts.

WHEN IS INFORMATION FROM THE CHART SHARED WITH OUTSIDERS?

Information in the charts is only accessible to the resident and their designate. In the case of a transfer or discharge, information about the resident is shared directly with the receiving facility or agency. Only information that is necessary for the safety and care of the resident should be shared. In some circumstances, information from inpatient stays in psychiatric hospitals is limited to a summary and recommendation of treatment. Copies of documents and other chart material can be shared only if the resident provides the facility with a signed/dated permission release request. For example, a resident is discharged from a hospital where there has been a neuropsychological evaluation. An overview/summary of this evaluation will generally be provided to the receiving facility. Additional information can be obtained with permission from the resident. In the case where a resident has had a previous nursing home placement, with a hospitalization in between, only a resident or guardian's signed/dated release can elicit chart or treatment information.

Another example: A resident is discharged to the community and has need of services from the Visiting Nurse Association (VNA), homemakers, and a day health center. All of these organizations may receive a 3-page referral with the necessary information to maintain their plan of care and assist in meeting their ongoing needs. Information written in the chart describing interactions between the social worker and the resident would not be provided unless this material is essential to the resident's ongoing care.

IS CONFIDENTIALITY AN ISSUE WITH REGARD TO FAX MACHINES?

It is important to remember in the age of the computer, with facsimile machines, telephone answering devices, and other electronic transmission of data that resident confidentiality needs to be maintained. The social worker should be providing minimum information in electronic transmissions. Follow-up phone calls to agencies to whom faxes are sent also assures proper transmission of information.

WHAT INFORMATION WOULD NOT BE PUT INTO THE CHART?

Social workers, at times, have access to information about residents that would be considered "sensitive." Some of this information is linked to the relationship of residents to their family members, some information is related to the resident's past. If the information is not particularly relevant to the resident's care and well-being in the facility, the social worker must use professional judgment of whether to record this in the chart. Here's an example: During obtaining background information for the social service history, a resident shares with the social worker that his affair (25 years earlier) with his daughter-in-law produced a child. The resident relates that he is somewhat embarrassed by this disclosure. He requests that the social worker leave out the detail of this child's conception, but not her existence as his daughter.

HOW IS CONFIDENTIALITY VIOLATED?

Maintaining confidentiality in a nursing facility can be as much of a problem as with any other institutional setting. There are several areas where confidentiality is dishonored:

- gossip;
- discussing a resident's case outside the facility, often using names;
- discussing resident's case with another resident's family;
- using material gathered from a resident's chart for printed material without seeking specific releases from the resident;
- allowing other residents or other resident's families to read or have access to records or charts that are not their own;
- discussing resident issues with other staff members or in public places, such as the elevator, nurses' stations, or other places where other residents or family members are present;
- providing information to other agencies or companies calling about the resident, that are not related to the discharge, transfer, or necessary services of the resident (e.g., a local pharmaceutical company wishes to have the names of residents suffering from osteoarthritis so that they can conduct a survey).

Violations of confidentiality are not always deliberate. They often occur, however, through the general negligence of staff to respect the importance of residents' right to have their records and life events private.

Social workers can help the staff understand their role in upholding confidentiality and the reasons that this is important. Through in-services and role modeling, social workers can provide the staff with support to prevent unnecessary disclosure of private material. In addition, social workers can advocate to protect residents from violations of their private records by not allowing surveys or research to be conducted upon the charts or records in the facility without the permission of residents involved.

In summary, social workers have a unique role in the facility with the residents, family and staff. By the nature of the profession, social workers have special access to a great deal of privileged information. Placement in a nursing home or adult resident for long-term care is equally complex and has financial, legal, and emotional aspects that must be carefully evaluated. All of these matters are fraught with stress for the older person who faces increased dependency at the hands of health providers, a spouse or children. All of these matters have ethical implications, sometimes requiring the social worker to assume the role of advocate for the client. The social worker is obligated to protect the rights of his or her clients in situations where these rights are being threatened (Nathanson & Tirrito, 1998, p. 19).

REFERENCES

Levy, C. (1993). *Social work ethics on the line.* New York: Haworth Press.
Nathanson, I. L, & Tirrito, T. T. (1998). *Gerontological social work.* New York: Springer Publishing Company, Inc.
Nursing Home Social Work Practice Standards.
Protecting the privacy of patients' health information: Summary of final regulation Health and Human Services. (2000). [On-line]. Available:http://www.hhs.gov/news/press/2000pres/00fsprivacy.html

CHAPTER THIRTY

Sexuality

HOW DOES THE TOPIC OF SEXUALITY AFFECT THE RESIDENT'S STAY IN THE NURSING FACILITY?

The topic of elder sexuality is one that the general public clouds with myths. Although we know the most intimate details of a resident's life, the area of sexuality rarely if ever is brought up as a routine issue. Nursing facilities are generally only concerned with resident sexuality if it presents a problem.

One newly admitted resident to a nursing facility recently commented to a social worker taking a social service history, "I don't mean to sound rude, but you've asked me about everything else in my life, except my sex life. Not that there is much." When the social worker, in a neutral tone, responded with, "What would you like tell me about that part of your life?" The resident replied, "Not much. I miss my wife, she was a great gal."

The social worker in this situation could have been shocked at the initial statement, even though it was prefaced with "I don't mean to sound rude." An inappropriate response of the social worker would probably not have helped the resident explore the issues around that statement. The resident appeared in this case to be trying to tell the social worker about his grief and loss around the death of his wife. He later told about missing the intimacy and the experiences he and his wife had shared through their 25 years of marriage.

Facility employees surveyed about resident sexuality in nursing homes, "expressed a need for proactive behavior from staff. They thought staff should understand the sexual needs of older people, especially their own feelings about sexuality. Many drew the line at staff encouraging sexual activities by residents" (Walker & Ephross, 1999, p. 103).

WHAT ARE SOME PROBLEMS AROUND THE LACK OF RESPECT FOR THE SEXUALITY OF OLDER ADULTS?

Sexuality also addresses the sexual identity of the person as a man or woman. Charlotte Eliopoulos (1993) stated that there are sometimes obvious signs of disregard to the elder's sexual identity through

Belittling the aged's interest in clothing, cosmetics, and hairstyles;
Dressing men and women residents of an institution in similar and asexual clothing;
Denying a woman's request for a female aide to bathe her;
Forgetting to button, zip, or fasten clothing when dressing the elderly;
Unnecessarily exposing aged individuals during examination or care activities;
Discussing incontinent episodes when the individual's involved peers are present;
Ignoring a man's desire to be clean and shaved before his female friend visits;
Not recognizing attempts by the aged to look attractive;
Joking about two aged persons' interest in and flirtation with each other (p. 112).

WHAT AREAS OF RESIDENT SEXUALITY ARE IMPORTANT?

Social workers should be aware of the myths that surround elder sexuality. Fran E. Kaiser (1996) has stated, "The persistent myth that aging and decline of sexual function inexorably are linked has led heath care providers to overlook one of the most important quality of life issues in older adults, that of sexuality. Sexuality encompasses sexual attitudes, behavior, practice and activity" (p. 100).

The social worker in the nursing facility can help address with both the staff and the residents that sexuality is a normal part of life. Sexuality also includes the intimacy of holding hands and having warmth and closeness with others. Hugs and kisses by people who care about the person often fulfill that basic need for human affection and sexuality. At the same time, nursing facilities cannot ignore the needs for privacy and intimacy of both married couples and residents who have special partners in their lives. Social workers can assist the facility in providing appropriate privacy for residents, without comment and judgment. "Consideration must be given to the sexual needs of older persons in institutional settings. Too often couples admitted to the same facility are not able to share a double bed, and frequently they are not even able to share the same room if they require different levels of care. It is unnatural, unreal, inhumane, and unfair to force a person to travel to another wing of a building to visit a spouse who has intimately shared 40, 50, or 60 years of their life" (Eliopoulous, 1993, p. 119).

ARE THERE MANY PROBLEMS WITH SEXUALITY IN NURSING FACILITY RESIDENTS?

Most residents of nursing facilities appear to be nonproblematic with respect to sexuality. In fact, many residents may be experiencing hyposexuality (reduced libido) as a result of being depressed or being on antidepressant medication.

There are residents, however, who provide challenges to nursing facilities because of how their sexuality activity is viewed. Generally a resident's sexuality comes to the attention of the staff when there is behavior that the nursing facility staff believes is inappropriate or labels "abnormal." In fact, the behavior that is not considered within "normal" limits in the facility may be a lifelong pattern that was viewed in the community as being acceptable. The observed sexual behavior may also be the result of a person's disease or medications.

Bonnie L. Walker and Paul H. Ephross (1999) studied staff attitudes towards elders' sexuality: "Respondents mostly thought people with dementia should not have sex though they were not in strong agreement on that issue. Regarding sexual abuse, the respondents believed staff are responsible for protecting residents and they recognized it is not always clear what is going on, consensual sex or abuse" (p. 104).

There are primarily three areas of observed problem behavior in the nursing facility:

1. Disinhibition—acting out:

   - confabulation
   - lewd talk
   - disrobing in public
   - physical advances toward staff, other residents
   - impulsiveness
   - inappropriate joking
   - exhibitionism

Some of the primary causes of this type of behavior are within the frontal lobe damage to the brain. In essence, the "stop" sign fails to restrict the behavior, or the indicator to stop comes on too late (Mitiguy, 1992).

2. Hypersexuality:

   - incessant talk about sexuality
   - disturbed sleep
   - increased appetite
   - propositioning staff and others

Primary causes of this type of behavior are associated with basal frontal or diencephalic lesions.

3. Undesirable behaviors with the staff:

   - grabbing at the caregiver's body, particularly the groin area, breasts, or buttocks
   - requesting staff to wash genital area when this activity could be easily completed by resident (this may be particularly requested of new, naive CNAs)

The causes of this behavior can be as simple as the body part of the caregiver being closest to the resident (from the position of the resident) when he or she needs attention. In other cases it may indicate a need for attention, that is, attention received for the behavior.

"Younger people can do with less touching; and theirs does not have the same significance. The older person feels closer to the end, perhaps partly gone. There is a loss of tactile sensation, a loss of companionship, a sense of deprivation. To touch is to regain contact with life, to feel alive" (Westheimer, 1987, p. 9). Social workers can assist the staff around these issues as they arise, helping to increase compassion, understanding, and appropriate behavioral responses.

It is important for the facility staff and caregivers to recognize that Alzheimer's Disease can also cause difficulties around sexuality. Koenig-Coste (1995) discusses this problem in terms of the disorientation personal relationships of the person with Alzheimer's Disease. Some suggestions offered for unwanted sexual behaviors for family members and caregivers:

- Divert attention;
- Be lovingly firm, "Please do not touch me;"
- Handle the situation delicately and privately;
- Address the situation immediately;
- Bathing or toileting may be assisted by someone of the same sex;
- Do not feel responsible for an inappropriate display of sexuality but:
- Be aware of your own body language and its message; and
- Discuss the situation with appropriate counsel (physician, Helpline counselor, social service department) (Koenig-Coste, p. 1).

WHAT HAPPENS WHEN TWO RESIDENTS IN THE FACILITY, ONE OF WHOM IS MARRIED (SPOUSE IN THE COMMUNITY) WISH TO HAVE AN INTIMATE RELATIONSHIP WITH ONE ANOTHER?

Although this question is not frequently an issue in a nursing facility, when the situation does arise, it can be very distressing for the caregiving team. There are a number of points which must be addressed:

- facility policy regarding private or privacy rooms for sexually active or intimate residents;
- the competency of both residents;
- the rights of the individual to freely associate;
- the rights of the roommates;
- confidentiality of records for resident;
- physician's orders;
- possible communicable illnesses/diseases.

One of the key points in determining how to view the residents' relationship is the issue of competency. The competent, consenting resident is obviously able to make decisions for herself. When the resident is not competent or has a guardian, the ability to consent or to make such decisions has been abrogated.

It is important for social workers to utilize professional judgment in these cases, to work with the residents, the team, the families, and the nursing facility administration. Some of these general issues can be brought forth for the ethics committee to address and discuss possible resolutions. Social workers can help facility staff with issues of sexuality through education and sensitivity.

REFERENCES

Eliopoulos, C. (1993) *Gerontological nursing.* Philadelphia: J. B. Lippincott Company.
Kaiser, F. E. (1996). Sexuality in the elderly. *Urologic Clinics of North America, 23,* 99–109.
Koenig-Coste, J. (1995). Alzheimer's and sexuality. *Alzheimer's Association Newsletter, 13*(2), 1–8.
Mitiguy, J. (1992). Neurologic damage to the anatomical substrate for sexual functioning. *Headlines, 3,* 4–5.
Walker, B. L., & Ephross, P. H. (1999). Knowledge and attitudes towards sexuality of a group of elderly. *Journal of Gerontological Social Work, 30*(1), 31–49.
Westheimer, R. (1987, October). Human sexuality means elders, too. *Provider,* 9–10.

PART EIGHT

Community Liaisons

CHAPTER THIRTY-ONE

Community Services

WHAT CAN COMMUNITY SERVICES DO FOR THE NURSING HOME RESIDENT?

Community services provide a huge selection resources a social worker can utilize to connect to residents' needs. There are several primary uses of community services:

- Community discharge planning;
- Services to residents in the nursing facility;
- Sources of networking for mutual referrals.

From the perspective of community services, most are thought to be linked to the process of the resident being discharged to the community. Social workers are most likely to think of services in umbrella groupings, such as

From the perspective of community services, many are linked to the process of the resident being discharged back home in the community. Social workers are most likely to think of services in umbrella groupings, such as

- Housing
  Elderly subsidized housing
  Assisted Living
  Foster Care
  Independent Housing
  Retirement communities
- Visiting Nurses (both public and private)
  Nurses
  Certified Home Health Aides
  Hospice
  Social Worker
  Physical Therapy,

Occupational Therapy, Speech Therapy
- Area Agencies on Aging
  Homemaker Services
  Chore Services
  Volunteer visitors
  Transportation
  Meal Sites
  Money managers
  Protective Services
  Elders at risk programs
  Case management
- Family Service Agencies
  Counseling for elders and families

213

Case management (at times)
Guardianship for elders in the community and at risk
• Councils on Aging
Transportation
Meals on Wheels

Access to other services in the area
Equipment
• Legal Services for elders
Guardianships, Power of Attorneys ·
Financial conflict resolution

Other services at various places include

• Adult Day Health Centers
• Senior Recreation Centers
• Independent case managers
• Emergency call systems
• Workshop or day treatment programs for residents with mental retardation or mental illness diagnosis
• Handicap renovation for homes/apartments (ramps, wheelchair accessible bathrooms, etc.)

Social work Departments in nursing facilities frequently keep resource books or lists of a range of services to elders in the community. An example of this was the *Guide to Long Term Care Alternatives in Massachusetts* that was updated annually and provided a wide range of residences for elders from assisted living apartments, foster care, adult day health centers, and congregate housing sites.

WHEN DO YOU UTILIZE THESE SERVICES?

When the resident and the team are discussing the home discharge, the social worker will begin to pull together a discharge plan that will assist the resident in maintaining his continuity of care. For example,

Miss Cora Appletree, 85, who had only a niece who lived out of state, was recovering from a fall and fractured left hip in Fresh Acres Nursing Home. Her rehabilitation was quite successful and the team felt she was ready to return to her Senior Housing apartment in the community. The social worker met with Miss Appletree to discuss the discharge. Miss Appletree stated that she wanted to use Phenomenal Care Nursing Services because "they had helped her in the past." The team had recommended that Miss Appletree have more physical therapy, a nurse to provide a dressing for the small but open area on her coccyx, and a home health aide to help with bathing. Miss Appletree had not been cooking well for herself before the fall. She had enjoyed the social hour at the facility. The social worker suggested Meals on Wheels initially upon discharge and then provided a referral for a meal site and transportation after her therapy was completed. Miss Appletree was also experiencing diminished eyesight. She stated she was having trouble making out her checks. The social worker made a referral for her to see a case manager to assess her needs for a "money manager" assistant.

The social worker helped to link Miss Appletree with the services that provided her with continuous care yet also provided her with independence.

WHAT COMMUNITY SERVICES COME INTO THE FACILITY?

There are a host of community services that enter the nursing facility. From Boy or Girl Scouts, to teen volunteers, to church ministries, to children's groups, the nursing facility can be a vibrant place as well as a part of the community. The services that specifically relate to social services are hospice, dialysis, and mental health counseling. All three of these services require physician orders. Although both dialysis and hospice tend to be more directly connected with nursing, social service will, as a member of the team, become a part of the treatment group. Helping the resident and the family accept a community service is an important role of the social worker. The social worker can also work closely with the team to provide the support needed in many of these situations. Mental health counseling is a service that comes into the facility from the community. (See Mental Health Consultants.)

HOW DOES HOSPICE WORK WITHIN THE NURSING FACILITY SETTING?

Although many people think of hospice for patients in the community, hospice also provides care and support to the dying in the nursing facility. Hospice providers contract with the nursing facility to provide services to residents. As this is a formal, financial contract, social workers need to be aware of the particular contracting agency in their facility. Hospice in the nursing facility, as in the community, provides

- Control of chronic pain
- Realism about death
- Staff support systems
- The "family" as the primary unit of caring

Hospice nurses assist the facility staff around the issues of caring for the dying resident. They offer support and realistic control for pain management, which can be, at times, a controversial issue in the nursing facility. Hospice offers counseling for the resident, the family, and also the staff as necessary. Hospice and the facility social worker work together to educate residents, families, and staff about the importance of the resident's comfort. Social workers can additionally support the hospice interventions as a part of the quality of life and dignity for the resident.

Social workers can find resources for themselves as well as family members in books such as Kenneth B. Wentzel's *To those who need it most . . . Hospice Means Hope,* Elisabeth Kubler-Ross' *Death: The Final Stage of Growth,* and *A Time to Grieve; Loss as a Universal Human Experience,* by Bertha G. Simos.

WHAT CAN YOU EXPECT FROM COMMUNITY SERVICES AT DISCHARGE?

Obviously this can vary from organization to organization. The social worker needs to clarify, however, before the resident's discharge, the who, what, when, and where questions, and relay this information to both the resident and the family or responsible party. This will ensure that the person returning home will anticipate the agency or service. In addition, some of the key components of good community service are

- Provision of the service on a timely basis (i.e., the service should be in the home on the day expected/promised)
- Services should be what was arranged (e.g., physical therapy or speech therapy or a thorough evaluation by that discipline)
- Follow-up for Protective Services or Elders at Risk, not merely a telephone call or a quick visit
- Charges or fees should be what was promised to the resident at discharge, with no hidden charges after the service was given

HOW DO COMMUNITY RESOURCES CONNECT REFERRALS TO THE FACILITY?

Community services also serve elders and families in the community who have not necessarily been in a nursing facility. If a resident requires nursing home care, there may be a time when these agencies will make the referral back to the facility. Positive feedback from the former residents of a nursing facility is an excellent recommendation for a nursing facility. In addition, appropriate discharge planning from the facility to the community agency will build good rapport and create a pleasant image of the nursing home to the public.

HOW DO ETHICAL ISSUES ARISE WITH COMMUNITY REFERRALS?

Community referrals should be based upon the service that will best meet the needs of the person, regardless of location, facility, or community. Choice, comparable services, and good previous experience should dictate which agency a social worker selects. Particular community agencies should not have inside priorities over other service providers. For example, a community agency should not attend the routine facility Medicare meetings where the staff discuss all the residents.

When it is the choice of the resident and family to have a community agency representative attend a resident care plan meeting, this can be helpful. In this case, the representative will be able to directly hear the specific needs of the resident and discuss how the agency can be helpful. Agency representatives can also provide handouts to residents and families that are helpful in the community connection process.

It is also necessary for the social worker, the resident, and family to discuss the needs of a resident returning to a particular assisted living center and determine what services are needed to continue the plan of care started in the nursing facility. Thompson's (1999) study of elders in community settings indicated "that many adult homes do not make available externally provided services nor do they refer residents to other sources of care when residents' needs change." Coordination can take place with the assisted living establishment, the health care provider, and insurer to provide the necessary treatment.

It is the social worker's professional responsibility to ensure that the resident has the optimum opportunity for choice of service agency. It is through experience and knowledge of local resources that the social worker can utilize a range of choices for discharging. It is important to always provide follow-up of services even if agencies are well known.

HOW DOES PPS AFFECT THE POST-NURSING HOME STAY?

On October 1, 2000, community services providers who receive payment through Medicare started billing through the Prospective Payment System. The system uses an instrument, Outcome and Assessment Information Set, or OASIS that is similar to the MDS. This instrument is used to determine the needs of the client upon referral as well as resuming care of a patient when the care is interrupted by an inpatient hospitalization. The implementation of this system is to increase accountability and focus the service. PPS and OASIS were tested in several home care provider state agencies before implementation. They were demonstrated at the time not to have a negative impact upon services. At this time, PPS is not being implemented for Medicaid recipients. It is important for the social worker, as the discharge planner, to be aware of the resources available and assist residents returning home to seek additional services if necessary.

REFERENCES

Guide to Long Term Care Alternatives in Massachusetts. (1998). Boston: Women's Educational and Industrial Union Home Care and Supportive Services, 356 Boylston Street, Boston, Massachusetts 02116.

Kubler-Ross, E. (1975). *Death the final stage of growth.* New York: Simon & Schuster Inc.

Thompson, J. M. (1999). Understanding variation in resident needs and services in homes for adults. *Social Work in Health Care, 30*(2), 49–63.

Wentzel, K. B. (1981). *To those who need it most, hospice means hope.* Boston: Charles River Books.

CHAPTER THIRTY-TWO

Ethnicity

HOW DOES ETHNICITY AFFECT RESIDENT PLACEMENT IN LONG-TERM CARE FACILITIES?

The issues of ethnicity are increasingly important in our changing American society. Estimates are that ethnicity and cultural differences in residents of long-term care facilities is representational of the population as a whole. As our population has become more diverse in urban and suburban areas, these changes have been reflected in the population of the local nursing homes. Ethnic groups have, in some large urban areas, developed specialized nursing homes that cater to specific ethnic groups, such as Italians, Greeks, Armenians, Chinese, or Germans. Religious groups, such as Baptists, Catholics, Hebrews, and Lutherans have also focused on the community/social needs of their members and developed nursing facilities that cater to their members. Although these facilities focus on the needs of these identified residents, admission to the facility cannot be limited because of antidiscriminations laws associated with federal and state funding laws.

Facilities located in areas where there are populations of Native Americans have been very few (Mercer, 1996). Native American communities have traditionally cared for their elders within the tribal systems and thus, when placement has occurred, the elder is often among those who do not speak the native language nor are they familiar with traditions surrounding caregiving. In some areas of the country there have been efforts to create institutions which provide care in a more culturally responsive way, such as the Navajo Nation nursing home in Chinle, Arizona, as studied by Mercer. She notes that elders are called "Grandparents" and there are many culturally specific traditions from personal care to dietary care, dying, and death (Mercer, 1996). She cites the important value of including the need for social workers and caregivers in nursing homes to check their cultural care practices. "It is easy to comprehend why elder Navajos who live off the reservation report loneliness, depression, and isolation, whereas the Grandparents at the nursing homes appeared to be content, satisfied, and 'at home.' Principles of care at the Chinle Nursing Home can be applied to other American Indian elders and nursing homes" (Mercer, 1996, p. 11).

These ethnic/cultural specific nursing homes offer residents and families the comfort of being surrounded by other residents who share language, religion, and/or culture-specific holidays. If the resident has recently immigrated to the U.S. from another country, the comfort of a familiar language and customs are often reassuring. Families also feel more comfortable in their choice of a facility, if it offers the resident a familiar atmosphere.

Not all residents seek a specialized nursing home, however, nor can they always locate a preferred ethnic, cultural, or racial facility. Residents and their families frequently select a nursing home based upon location for easy family visits. Others choose a facility that meets the physical needs of the resident without concern for the cultural or religious aspects.

DOES ETHNICITY, RACE, OR RELIGIOUS AFFILIATION AFFECT THE RESIDENT'S ADJUSTMENT TO THE FACILITY?

Yes. Obviously the importance of ethnicity, religious affiliation, racial or cultural background can vary significantly from resident to resident. Based upon their prior life experiences, entrance into a nursing facility can be a continuation of the older person's past experiences with institutional settings. All nursing homes share common threads of a total institutional setting, such as being a medical setting, institutional rules, shared spaces, institutionally prepared meals, and so forth. A resident's previous life experience with bureaucracy will probably be relevant as well.

Residents for whom English is a second language may have a wide range of reactions of acclimation to the setting. Those who speak English very well, and who have been become acclimated to U.S. culture, may not need or desire an ethnically specialized facility. On the other hand, for residents who do not speak English, for whom the United States culture has been a relatively new experience, an ethnically appropriate facility may help the transition.

Perhaps the most important components in the adjustment process of minority groups are the resiliency of the older person in her adaptability, the degree to which the family has adjusted and accepted change, and the degree to which the facility is able to support the integrity of the residents and their affiliations. It is also important for the social worker to be aware of the issues presenting, and assess the resident's needs within the context, without ethnocentric biases.

HOW DOES SOCIAL SERVICE ASSIST WITH THE ADJUSTMENT OF CULTURALLY, ETHNICALLY, RELIGIOUSLY, AND RACIALLY VARIED RESIDENTS?

Social workers have the role of helping those who are unable to speak the language obtain translation as it is needed to ensure that their needs will be met within the nursing facility and they are provided with an opportunity to access their rights:

- residents who speak another language have a copy of resident rights in a language that they can read;

- residents who do not speak English need to have a way to communicate their needs to the staff;
- access to a translator on staff;
- a written communication board, utilizing pictures as well as translations;
- family member translation;
- access to a translator from the community;
- residents should be free to and encouraged to continue to practice their religious beliefs as long as doing so does not interfere with other residents;
- residents who have particular dietary requests should be accommodated and they should not be denied full benefits of a healthy diet because of these preferences;
- enhance resident and family access to services available in the facility.

Social workers can help other residents and staff become more tolerant and supportive of diversity through education programs, and encouraging communication between all residents and their family members of the facility.

The facility can enhance the knowledge of diversity through uniting residents, families, and staff in the positive aspects of diversity. Providing written literature (pamphlets) about different groups, and arranging times when residents, families, and staff can share particular holidays with particular foods and entertainment can enhance acceptance of diversity.

In many cultures, elders are viewed with a great deal of respect, and this respect is conveyed in numerous small ways, for example, in handing an elder an object, the Chinese display of respect is to use two hands. To hand a person an object with a single hand is a show of disrespect. Social service can be observant of these differences and help moderate any miscommunication that may occur between the resident and a caregiver.

WHAT ARE SOME OF THE PROBLEMS WITH DIVERSITY IN THE NURSING FACILITY?

Some of the difficulties that arise in having a diverse resident population are

- inadequate staff training around racial, ethnic, or cultural variations;
- language barriers that are inadequately met by the facility in trying to meet the care needs of the resident;
- cultural inconsistencies that are not addressed by the facility;
- lack of respect for residents' ethnicity, cultural practices;
- racism, specifically differential treatment of residents based upon their race or ethnic background;
- poor communication with family members by the facility.

Social workers can help increase communications through development of specific interventions with families and residents as they are identified. One of the key components of increasing adjustment is through the use of translators. For example,

Mr. and Mrs. K. were a Chinese-American couple who had been placed in a local nursing facility by their son who, because of his extensive, intense work schedule could no longer care for the couple in his home. It was a very difficult decision for him because of the historical cultural values of his parents' country that dictated eldest sons care for their parents. The close proximity of the facility to his home, however, made this an accepted choice for his family. Both the residents were relatively new to the U.S.; they did not speak any English. According to the son, their mental status was impaired as well, making translation even in their own language difficult. The couple were the only Mandarin speaking residents in the facility. The facility did not have any Chinese speaking CNAs or nurses. Initially, though Mr. K.'s son's wife visited daily to see her in-laws, multiple interventions were necessary to ensure their care and comfort. The speech therapist developed a simple pictorial/Chinese language translation board to help the residents and the staff address day-to-day needs. A family member was also requested by the facility to be "available" to provide routine translations as necessary and accompany either parent to medical appointments. After several months, it became apparent that the family was becoming increasingly inconsistent in their visits and that they and the residents were noncompliant with the facility smoking requests (by smoking in the residents' room). A family meeting was held with an outside translator present to enhance communication. This meeting helped to clarify some of the issues presented.

Social workers can also assist staff with diversity issues through formal in-services. Staff in-services can highlight the need to address cultural, ethnic, or religious diversity and preferences during care or dietary preferences. Recognition of residents' differences can be creatively handled in a variety of ways (e.g., Family Council members can provide a forum of information or even an event centered around a religious holiday).

WHAT ARE THE PROBLEMS WITH DIVERSITY IN STAFF?

Discrimination and intolerance of others can be a problem between residents and staff. Although diversity of the community at large is reflected in many areas of the nursing facility staff, the variation of cultures and/or race can present problems dating from when intolerance was an acceptable practice. Segregation was a fact of life for many years in this country, as well as in others. The result of these practices can be strong, open, residual prejudice.

In addition, these attitudes can also be based in a long history of the individual's biased, negative view toward certain groups of people. Caregiving requires individuals to rely upon one another in circumstances that are less than desirable—the basis for the need of a nursing facility placement: physical ailments or incapacity. For elders who have harbored discrimination and prejudice in their community life, adapting to caregivers who are different from them can present a very real challenge.

Some discrimination toward staff can be a manifestation of the physical disorders, such as dementia or hearing losses. Regardless of the basis, it is important for the social worker to be aware of problems that the staff encounter in caring for residents who are particularly prejudiced, and assist in resolution.

For example, the social worker might observe the successful care of a resident by a particular CNA. If this lessens the angry outbursts and tensions, regularly pairing the resident with this particular CNA might be a solution.

Social workers can provide direct counseling for the resident who is actively, verbally prejudiced, and encourage him to accept care. If the resident's prejudice is a product of a lifetime and compromised by dementia, however, nursing assignments need to reflect and address this problem. Forcing a resident to be compliant, or not addressing the issue as a problem can lead to potentially abusive or neglectful situations. Some staff are resistant to making accommodations, calling adjustments "spoiling." Increasing a resident's cooperation and decreasing the tension around care issues is not inappropriate catering. Meetings with the resident, family, and the nursing staff can help to focus on these circumstances and create an acceptable solution. Recognition of serious conflict and an appropriate response to this problem creates a calmer atmosphere and ultimately is a win-win situation for everyone.

> There are a number of themes running through all the research on minority groups. Members of minority groups generally receive lower incomes and have fewer job opportunities than do members of the dominant group. First-generation immigrants in particular are required to take the least preferred jobs at the lowest salaries. Members of a minority group generally have shorter life expectancy up to age 65 than do dominant group members, but at some point beyond that age they enjoy a longer life expectancy. Because of past discrimination, members of minority groups usually receive smaller retirement incomes, are more likely to live with extended relatives, are less likely to be able to maintain independent living in the later years and are generally less well educated than the dominant group. They often receive fewer government services than the dominant group. The rationalization often heard is that the families of minority groups are very tightly integrated and that they consider it important to look after their older members. This rationalization begs the question since if the government provided needed services to older members of minority groups it would probably not be necessary for their families to assume this responsibility. (Cox, 1996, p. 76)

In summary, diversity in the nursing facility is a reflection of the community as well as society in the United States. The ethnic patterns in communities will continue to change and shift for both residents and staff. It is important for the nursing home social worker to be aware of ethnically related caregiving values and behaviors in planning for elder care. Their role can be pivotal in an elder's comfort of cultural continuity and the social worker can advocate for residents and family members within larger systems of care.

Social workers can continue to expand their knowledge base about ethnicity in multiple arenas. They can attend local continuing education conferences about the elderly and ethnicity. Some may find information on the Internet, or through their local area agency on aging (AAA). Many utilize print professional resources such as Browne and Broderick's (1994) article, "Asian and Pacific Islander," in *Social Work*, Burnnette's (1999) article on custodial grandparents in Latino families, also in *Social Work*. Nursing home social workers should be particularly sensitive to individual cultural variations in discharge planning with families and residents. Delgado and Tennstedt (1997) discuss the Puerto Rican family structure where sons are the primary caregivers. And there is also variation within the Hispanic community as is discussed by Castex (1994) in her article "Providing services to Hispanics/Latino populations; profiles in diversity."

REFERENCES

Browne, C., & Broderick, A. (1994). Asian and Pacific Island elder issues for social work practice and education. *Social Work, 39*(5), 252–259.

Burnnette, D. (1999). Custodial grandparents in Latino families: Patterns of service use and predictors of unmet needs. *Social Work, 44*(1), 22–25.

Castex, G. M. (1994). Providing services to Hispanics/Latino populations; profiles in diversity. *Social Work, 5*(39), 288–296.

Cox, H. G. (1996). *Later life: The realities of aging.* New Jersey: Prentice Hall.

Delgado, M., & Tennstedt, S. (1997). Puerto Rican sons as primary caregivers of elderly parents. *Social Work, 42*(3), 125–135.

Mercer, S. O. (1996). Navajo elderly people in a reservation nursing home: Admission predictors and culture care practices. *Social Work, 41*(2), 181–200.

CHAPTER THIRTY-THREE

Funeral Arrangements

HOW DOES THE NURSING FACILITY SOCIAL WORKER BECOME INVOLVED IN FUNERAL ARRANGEMENTS?

There are several points of entry for this topic for the nursing facility social worker:

- at the time of admission, chart face sheets frequently ask for advance arrangements;
- applications for Medicaid (Medi-Cal, Mass Health, etc.) ask about prepaid funeral arrangements;
- when a resident has planned an anatomical gift prior to admission;
- an unexpected death in the facility where a funeral home has been not specified and there is not family member available;
- a family member or resident makes a request of information from the social worker.

Funeral arrangements, as a topic, are often difficult for people in our culture to discuss. Indeed, for many, the issues of dying, death, and the process of making decisions around a person's death are almost taboo. Even families, when faced with the terminal illness of a loved one, can put off making arrangements. The social worker can address these issues in a manner that is helpful and supportive to both the resident and the family.

During the admissions process, social workers can address the topic of funeral arrangements as a general issue. The simple question, "Have you, or the resident, a preference for a funeral home?" can open the door to discussions of end life decisions as well as reveal tensions over illness, loss, and dying. Previous losses and prior funeral arrangements can be discussed with the family to prepare them for making some decisions. Although some individuals consider this "morbid," the preplanning is much easier than trying to cope with making arrangements as well as dealing with the death of a loved one. For example,

Miss Alberta Collins, 75, had been at Sunny Acres for 8 months, when she was diagnosed with a rapid growing cancer. Prior to her admission, she had spent a

lifetime being admitted to and discharged from state psychiatric hospitals for her primary diagnosis of schizophrenia. A niece, Valerie Smith, had held temporary guardianship at one point, just prior to her admission to the facility and had maintained a distant relationship. Miss Collins's condition had suddenly deteriorated and she was hospitalized one Monday. By the following Thursday her condition had declined further and she was taken off the respirator, and shortly thereafter, passed away. The hospital called both the niece and the nursing facility looking for directions regarding her funeral. The resident chart did not contain any designated arrangements. Dismayed by this information, Ms. Smith realized, belatedly, that unless she provided the funds, the state would provide a "pauper's burial" for her aunt.

The social worker can assist the family to address the funeral arrangement issues by discussing the Medicaid application where prepaid funeral arrangements can be an allowable expense. Families often choose to create a prepaid funeral at the point of application or just prior to the application process, as this may count as a general "spend-down" of a resident's assets. According to the National Funeral Directors Association (2000), more than 7 million living Americans have prearranged their funerals.

Social workers who work in facilities where a resident without family or friends has passed away, may be put in the position of discussing the funeral arrangements with a local funeral director. She will be dealing with the basics of the funeral and making decisions that a family would have to consider. Gravesites are unmarked for state subsidized burials.

WHAT ARE THE COSTS OF A FUNERAL?

The costs of a funeral and burial, insurance benefits, as well as an obituary may be part of the discussion. Funerals in 1999 averaged to be around $5778.16 according to the National Funeral Directors Association (2000). Costs can vary significantly, however, according to the type of funeral service and whether the choice is burial or cremation. Caskets can vary in price from the $595.00 model (cloth covered corrugated fiberboard) to the $7,000.00 model made of solid copper. There are often standard costs that will not vary much, such as the mandatory (legal) preparation of the body, the costs of opening a grave, the mandatory liner of the gravesite, and closure of the grave. Obviously the cost of grave markers can vary significantly as well. Other variables in the cost of the funeral are the services of the funeral director, the printed material, the automotive services, and use of the facilities for the wake.

WHAT ARE THE COSTS FOR CREMATION?

The costs for cremation are significantly less than those for a funeral. Direct cremation costs can range from $880–$1,000. Rentals for chapel, private viewing, memorial, and graveside services are from $750 and up. There are also various options for disposition, including mailing out of country, and arranging the scattering. Residents and family members should seek specific information for cremation from cremation organizations throughout the country and Canada.

ARE THERE TYPICAL RESOURCES TO PAY FOR A FUNERAL IF A PREPAID FUNERAL IS CONTRACTED?

Yes. Resources to help with the cost of the funeral come from a variety of sources. Some residents have paid or maintained life insurance policies, some have insurance through their pension programs, and others have put aside a certain bank account for the purpose of burial. Social Security also offers a tiny contribution of a $255.00 "lump sum death benefit." The funeral director can be of assistance in claiming of benefits when the resident does not have a family.

WHAT HAPPENS TO A RESIDENT'S WISH TO DONATE HIS OR HER BODY FOR ANATOMICAL RESEARCH?

Social workers also can provide assistance in maintaining the wishes of a resident who has requested his body to be an anatomical gift. The person may wish to donate an organ or he may wish to have the body used for further medical investigation of disease. It is important in these cases that the resident's body be transported to the correct location. This specific information should be recorded on the face sheet of the resident's chart. If the resident has made arrangements, the social worker should provide this specific data in the written transfer referral information when the resident is sent to the hospital or transferred to another facility. As with all other advance directives, there should be routine confirmation of these wishes.

WHAT IS THE POLICY REGARDING A DEATH IN THE NURSING FACILITY?

Social workers should be aware of the facility policy around the death of a resident at the facility. Often, there are set protocols that help with addressing how the remains of the person are transported out of the facility. If upon occasion, the body must remain in the nursing facility for an extended time, there are arrangements for temporary storage.

In some facilities, the person who has expired is left in the bed, the nursing staff performs the postmortem duties, and awaits the funeral home to remove the body. Curtains are drawn between the beds in the room and the deceased is provided "privacy."

In other facilities, the resident who has died is taken to a predesignated storage room (often close to an exit door) after postmortem care. These types of facility policies may also include excluding residents on the unit from seeing the remains of the resident being transported and discourage conversation about the death.

The social worker needs to advocate for residents and staff to have the opportunity to express their feelings about the loss and to mourn. This may include:

- Allowing residents, or staff, if they wish, to view and visit briefly with the resident who has died before the undertaker from the funeral home arrives;
- Grieve for the loss of a friend and perhaps roommate;
- Express their sympathies to the bereaved family members;
- Participate in funerals or memorial services;
- Providing policy and system to collect the resident's belongings to give to the family, avoiding the plastic bag lumping of clothing and personal effects;
- Noting what items, if any, have been taken by the funeral home from the facility;
- Providing opportunities for residents, families and friends to donate gifts or memorial funds in the name of the resident(s) who have lived and passed on at the facility.

In summary, social workers in nursing facilities are in prime positions to help residents, families, and staff around both the advanced directive issue as well as the emotional impact of death. Addressing advanced directive choices, such as the selection of a funeral home, helps to bring up important policy issues and allows the family and resident to recognize the care and concern the facility staff has for all aspects of a resident's stay.

REFERENCE

National Funeral Directors Association. (2000). [On-line]. Available: http://www.nfda.org/resources/99gpl.html

PART NINE

Problems and Solutions

CHAPTER THIRTY-FOUR

Troubles in Paradise

In describing their work, the social workers most often used the term advocate, as in "You end up being an advocate for the resident a lot," or "They see me as their advocate" . . . most prominent was the notion of advocating to staff particularly nurses and nurses' aides. (Reinardy, 1999)

Problems in the long-term care facility are not necessarily always present. Like other work settings, however, difficulties among staff members are not unusual. Though generally manageable, issues within the setting take time to resolve and remediate. The following are highlighted areas where the social worker can encounter some work-based challenges.

WHAT ARE SOME OF THE POWER AND CONTROL ISSUES?

As with any formal employment setting, there are the formal identified roles that an organizational chart outlines and then there are the operational organizational charts, that never appear on paper. It is important for the social worker to recognize and work within both the "seen" organizational structure as well as the "unseen." Again, as with any company, power and control can be orchestrated from seemingly innocuous positions such as the medical records person, or the office business manager who handles the accounts. Power comes when the normally designated person to the position is either absent, weak, or ineffectual, and another person sees this opportunity to gain power and control. As a result, formal organizational chart designations can become skewed or lopsided in day-to-day operations.

It is important for the social worker to clearly identify, prioritize, and delineate assignments for any "extra" roles in the facility. The effort to become a "team player" can often encourage job overlap, such as answering the facility telephone during an off time or responding to a resident's call light. On the other hand, the evening nurse on a unit could provide the extra "social work" support to a resident who expresses a desire to talk about a loss or relationship problem.

Team members should be encouraged to support one another; at the same time, they also need to shoulder their own roles and jobs within the facility. The social worker can also help by setting realistic limits for work and duties assigned, such as, "I'd love to help you with the phone, but I need to run my resident group this afternoon." Presenting realistic, concrete responses to inappropriate assignments helps social workers to educate others in the facility of their roles.

WHAT IS THE "MARTYR SYNDROME"?

Regardless of the facility, the discipline, or the time period, there are always the folks who will martyr themselves for the "cause." These are the employees who stay all hours of the night to put the "facility in order." In contrast to those workers who exit the nursing home with the pencil in the air, at precisely 4:00 PM or 5:00 PM every evening, the martyrs are ever-present on weekends, late evenings, from 7:00 AM or earlier in the morning to 9:00 PM at night. Their knowledge of residents, staffing, current regulations are extensive. They may share this important information, but generally it is provided on an "as needed basis." These folks can actually carry on like this for years, as long as the administration provides the appropriate feedback, "we need you," the martyrs keep up their eternal vigil.

Social service should avoid becoming the facility martyr. For obvious reasons it is not a healthy role. Moreover it is a relationship with residents and staff that is not realistic. Occasional late nights are not in the same category as becoming the facility martyr. If you have concerns about whether you are a facility martyr, you might consider answering the following questions:

Yes ☐ No ☐ 1. Do you stay late in the facility one hour or more every day?

Yes ☐ No ☐ 2. Do you frequently work weekend days without equivalent time off or rotation?

Yes ☐ No ☐ 3. Do you refuse personal social activities because you feel that you need to be available to work?

Yes ☐ No ☐ 4. Do you refuse opportunities to go to conferences or continuing education programs because you feel that you are "missing too much work"?

Yes ☐ No ☐ 5. Do you take work home on a regular basis, three to four nights a week?

Yes ☐ No ☐ 6. Do your fellow employees tell you that you work too much?

Yes ☐ No ☐ 7. Do you think that you are the only one who can do the "job" right?

Yes ☐ No ☐ 8. Does your family complain that they never see you?

Yes ☐ No ☐ 9. In your spare time do you think or worry about the work you have left to do at the facility?

Yes ☐ No ☐ 10. Are your social contacts primarily with the staff at the facility?

If you answered yes to more than three of these questions, you might well be on your way to becoming a formal martyr. It is very important to prioritize your work life and your personal life. Work, is just that, "work." In order to provide residents with your best, you cannot be only one-sided, that is, only "the social worker." Take some time to develop different interests and hobbies. Provide yourself with outlets that are constructive and positively reinforce you as a truly unique person.

HOW ARE NURSING FACILITIES DYSFUNCTIONAL?

Dysfunction can occur in any workplace, from educational institutions to bottle factories. Workplaces can generate cooperation as well as discord among employees. Dysfunctional situations do occur in nursing facilities, though not often, and the range of maladaptive behavior(s) can be quite broad, from mismatched employee skills and job assignments to the extreme—deliberate malfeasance.

As with many other employment situations and large corporations, nursing facilities are frequently stretching their employee efforts with increasing workloads. This can result in varied responses and adaptive behavior problems. For example,

> *Marli K., a nurse at Sunny Acres, was recently promoted to the position of charge nurse of the Medicare unit. A shy, quiet young person, Marli K. had only worked at the facility for about 3 months when a round of administrative layoffs left the unit two nurses short. Marli K. was flattered by the sudden promotion, but the demands of the job entailed assigning a group of "street savvy," older CNAs to their work. It was a difficult task, and Marli K.'s strategy for dealing with the CNAs difficult behavior was to avoid confrontation and to busy herself with paperwork. When residents complained that their bells were not being answered, or their care was rough, Marli K. would try to deflect the complaints with soothing statements like, "Oh, they didn't mean to do that," or vaguely respond, "I'll speak to them." She never approached the CNAs about their work with residents, however, and rarely left the nursing station.*

The social worker who observed this situation wanted to respond. He found there were several choices:

- He could remain detached from the situation and problems because "it was a nursing department issue."
- He could attempt to quietly counsel Marli K. and the CNAs about their roles with one another and the residents.
- He could meet with the management of the facility, the nursing supervisor, the director of nurses or the assistant director of nurses and discuss his concerns openly.

Which choice might you make? Your choice might be based upon your role, your perceived role, your skills as a mediator, and the level of dysfunction of the setting. Whatever your choice, your role in the facility as a social worker will create an impact upon the staff and the residents.

WHAT IS THE DELEGATION SYNDROME?

Delegation is an interesting phenomenon in nursing facilities that can come from any number of sources on the team. As with other industries and bureaucracies, job descriptions often have a tag-on sentence that states, "and duties as otherwise assigned." This brief statement provides the cover for the administration to assign staff to duties that are not specifically stated in the job description. Job descriptions are most often sweeping outlines of a position in the facility. They frequently leave a great deal to individual administrative discretion.

There are of course limits to what a social worker can be assigned to do. The social worker, even those who are doubly certified or licensed, cannot suddenly switch and give out medications, physically care for residents, or change dressings. At the same time, there are a multitude of clerical, business functions from the process of admissions to discharge that can be assigned to the social work department through delegation.

WHO DELEGATES? HOW DOES THE SOCIAL WORKER KNOW WHAT IS A PART OF THE JOB AND WHAT IS NOT?

Delegation of duties and assignments can be a very haphazard process. In most facilities, the person's direct superior assigns work; in the social worker's case this is generally the facility administrator. The administrator can request volunteer assistance from members of the staff, or she can literally assign specific duties to the group based upon the needs of the facility.

The additional assignment of duties can occur when the nursing home is going through the stresses and strains of employee changes or shortages of staff. In these cases the key duties of one department are necessarily absorbed and shared by others. It is expected and anticipated; the rearranged assignments will revert back to their original source once the facility is again fully staffed. This delegation process encompasses the notion of teamwork and provides and supports the continuity necessary to meet the needs of the residents and families.

The social worker needs to be familiar with the facility social work job description. As new or additional duties are delegated, it is important for the social worker to compare these functions to the job description and determine if they fall under the umbrella of the "other duties as assigned." If there are small components of the social work department facility duties that are not included in the job description that the social worker performs, this does not mean there is a problem. On the other hand, if the social worker is spending more than 50–60% of his time in performing business office duties and admissions work, then we could certainly view this as problematic. Blurring duties and taking on additional responsibilities can quickly or eventually interfere with the social worker's ability to provide services and perform as a social worker for the facility.

The job of purchasing resident clothing, for instance, is frequently assigned to social workers for a variety of reasons. This time-consuming task has little to do with therapeutic alliance of social worker and client. However, having residents properly clothed does help residents' psychological sense of well-being and self-esteem. It can also be viewed as a social service problem when families are not providing resources for the resident. The social worker can utilize this concrete need to network with first staff, and then families, to encourage and to engage them in purchasing necessary needed items for the resident. It should not be the primary position of the social worker to directly purchase clothing or arrange for shopping trips for the residents. For example,

In the Gray Swallow Nursing Facility, Sonia Peters, the new facility social worker, was told by the administrator her job was to order clothing as needed for residents, arrange for hearing evaluations and label dentures and glasses with a special tool. Sonia was angered at this request, feeling it was "not her job." An MSW with other long-term care facility experience, she felt her time was not being well used in this capacity. Through a process of both creative thinking (the facility had many involved family members), and the need to assist the resident, Sonia devised several facility systems to respond to the needs of the residents as well as empower family members to take an active role in the life of their resident. Families of residents with specific needs were contacted and provided with written referrals or instructions about labeling residents' belongings. A clothing provider agreed to provide services, such as measuring and work with families around ordering. Only to those residents who did not have any family or friends available did Sonia directly provide care. Even this direct care, though, was a joint effort with the nursing staff and the facility bookkeeper. Thus she met the needs of the residents without redefining the facility social work position.

It is important for the social worker to advocate for the social service position in the facility as it was designed. Social work as a discipline is not always clearly identified and understood by the public at large, and these blurred concepts can be carried through to the nursing facility as well. Concrete assignments and procedures often gain more recognition by staff and administration; as a result, the delegation of nonsocial work functions can take place. If the social worker finds that there are too many nonsocial service functions being delegated or assigned, she must pursue the issue with the facility administrator.

There are many facilities where the team members complement each other in skill and expertise. In these settings, the social worker can function in her given role, facilitate emotional growth, and assist in generating a place where residents and their families feel comfortable and receive excellent care. Indeed, many social workers and even residents could call these facilities paradise.

REFERENCE

Reinardy, J. R. (1999). Autonomy, choice, and decision making: How nursing home social workers view their role. *Social Work in Health Care, 29*(3), 59–77.

PART TEN

Standardized Forms

Initial Social Service History and Assessment Form

There are multiple forms that have been designed to gather information about the history of a resident during the initial admission. These are adequate to obtain information about the resident, however, all forms limit spontaneous information and many forms do not necessarily reflect material that is requested for the MDS. The use of these forms can be

- at initial admission as an informational gathering tool;
- for a short-term admission in conjunction with the MDS information;
- replacement of an independent social service history.

Chart Location: These forms can be found in the Social Service section of the chart. The social service history should immediately follow the pre-admission note(s) and precede any follow-up notes.

SOCIAL SERVICE HISTORY
INITIAL ASSESSMENT

Date of Admission: Source of Payment upon Admission:

Name: Sex: M ❐   F ❐   Marital Status: S M W D

Ethnicity: Date of birth:

Place of birth: Religion:

US citizen: Yes ❐ No ❐   Date of immigration:

Languages spoken: Is English understood: Yes ❐ No ❐

Source of this information: Chart ❐   Resident ❐   Other: ❐

Diagnoses:

Reason for placement:
Expectations/Goals of this placement:

Brief physical description of the resident (include ambulatory status):

History of illness and/or accident/injury:

Previous hospitalizations:

Origin of family:
Parents' names:
If deceased, when and cause:
Siblings' names, addresses, phone numbers:

Closest siblings or friends to person:
Education:
Schools attended and last grade completed:

Military Service:

Occupation(s):
  Where:
  Type of work:
  How long:
  Date of retirement:
Names of spouse(s) (indicate whether still living):
  Dates of marriage(s):
  Description of relationship(s):

If spouse is no longer living, indicate adjustment of resident to living alone:

Children: Yes ☐   No ☐
Children's names, ages, addresses and phone numbers:

Are any children deceased?

Describe personally; include psychosocial relationships with family, friends and whether these have changed:

Describe resident's use of spiritual comfort:

Describe mood, emotional status, and mental status, past and present; discuss whether resident has changed:

Ability to read: Yes ☐   No ☐
Write: Yes ☐   No ☐
Tell time: Yes ☐   No ☐
Has the resident ever been treated for depression, substance abuse, or a mental disorder? If so when, where, and with what response?

Is the resident presently receiving psychoactive medications? If yes, list below and note effectiveness. Note length of time, if known.

Describe the best approaches for working with the resident:

Resident strengths or skills:

Discharge plans:

Social service goals for this placement:

Information completed by: Date:

Pre-Admission Screening Scenario

OBRA Pre-Admission screening is required when

Any new admission to a nursing facility occurs.

Any in-patient *psychiatric* hospitalization occurs.

A nursing home resident is discharged to the community and decompensates, necessitating readmission to a nursing facility. At that time, a new level I screening by the home care/hospital will trigger the PASSAR process.

OBRA Pre-Admission screening is not required when

A nursing home resident transfers from one nursing facility to another. The *sending* facility should include a copy of the most recent OBRA screening with the accompanying paperwork.

A nursing home resident is sent to a hospital for *medical* reasons. The 20-day bed-hold practice often utilized by discharge planners does not enter into consideration. This scenario also includes residents who are discharged to a different nursing facility after a medical admission. It is incumbent on the *receiving* facility to contact the previous nursing home or the OBRA offices for a copy of the most recent OBRA screening.

A nursing home resident is approved for a 90-day stay and *has* received an OBRA/PASARR during that time period. No additional screening will be required if a conversion to long-term nursing home level of care is requested. Those residents admitted to an in-patient psychiatric hospital at or before the 90-day mark will fall under scenario II.

In order to ensure compliance with this federally mandated process, all hospital, nursing facility, and home care staff persons are encouraged to review each admission/discharge carefully.

IDENTIFICATION SCREENING FOR NONRECIPIENTS WAIVING LTC SCREENING

This form is to be completed only for those individuals who meet the eligibility criteria for nursing facility services as described in 106 CMR 456.251 through 456.266.

Provider Information Section		Recipient Information Section	
Provider Name & Address		Recipient's Name & Address	Sex
			❑ M ❑ F
Provider's Telephone No.	Provider No.	Date of Birth	Recipient ID No.
( )			

Section I. Identification

1. Does the individual have a documented diagnosis or treatment history of any of the following major mental disorders?
   - ❑ Schizophrenia
   - ❑ Major Affective Disorder
   - ❑ Atypical Psychosis
   - ❑ Paranoia
   - ❑ Schizoaffective Disorder
   - ❑ None of the above

2. Does the individual have a documented diagnosis or treatment history of mental retardation, developmental disability, or a related condition?
   ❑ Yes ❑ No

3. Does the individual exhibit any evidence of a major mental illness?
   ❑ Yes ❑ No

4. Has the individual ever received inpatient or outpatient psychiatric treatment?
   ❑ Yes ❑ No

5. Has the individual received services for mental retardation, developmental disability, or a related condition from an agency that serves the mentally retarded, the developmentally disabled, or both?
   ❑ Yes ❑ No

6. Does the individual exhibit any evidence that may indicate mental retardation, developmental disability, or a related disorder?

    ❐ Yes   ❐ No

    (If you have answered *"No"* to all of the above, skip *Section II* and go on to *Section III.*)

Section II. Exemptions for Mental Illness Only (Complete only if you answered *"Yes"* to at least one question in *Section I.*)

Does the individual meet any of the following conditions? (Check those that apply.)

- ❐ Alzheimer's disease or other dementia (requires supportive documentation)
- ❐ Comatose
- ❐ Ventilator-dependent
- ❐ Brain-stem level functioning
- ❐ Severe chronic obstructive pulmonary disease
- ❐ Severe Parkinson's disease
- ❐ Severe Huntington's disease
- ❐ Severe amyotrophic lateral sclerosis
- ❐ Severe congestive heart failure
- ❐ Convalescent care not to exceed 30 days following acute hospital stay
- ❐ Terminal illness certified by physician (less than six-month prognosis)

Section III. Certification

Based on the above findings, I certify that (check one):

- ❐ There is no indication of mental illness, mental retardation, or developmental disability.
- ❐ Mental illness is indicated, but individual meets one of the exemptions in Section II.
- ❐ Mental illness, mental retardation, or developmental disability is indicated and referral has been made to the appropriate agency for assessment.

Signature: _____   Date: _____

Title: _____

REFUSAL OF PREADMISSION SCREENING FOR NONRECIPIENTS

I, _____, hereby acknowledge that I have been made aware of the opportunity for, but have refused, a preadmission screening by the Department or its contracted agency prior to entering _____ facility as a private-paying resident. I understand that I will be subject to screening by the Department or its contracted agency if at any time I apply for Medical Assistance (Medicaid) reimbursement for my nursing facility stay.

I also understand that if the screening performed at the time of application for Medicaid indicates that my care needs do not justify continued stay in a nursing facility, my transfer from the facility may be required, and reimbursement by Medicaid will not be authorized.

_____

Patient's Signature

_____

Responsible Party's Signature

_____

Witness's Signature

(A copy of this form must be forwarded with the Long Term Care Assessment Form to the Department or its contracted agency at the time of application for Medicaid. A copy must be included in the permanent nursing facility record.)

Notices for Transfer or Discharge

Nursing facilities have all developed their own notices to inform residents of proposed transfers or discharges. Written notices must be given to the resident and their designee 30 days before the proposed transfer or discharge, or in limited circumstances, as soon as practicable before the action.

All notices are written in 12-point type or larger. Notification includes the name of the facility, the transfer or discharge decision, the place where the resident is going, the reason(s) for the transfer, and both the date of the notice and the date of the proposed transfer. Included in all notifications are the resident's rights and a form describing their right to appeal the facility decision and agencies, addresses, and telephone numbers to help. Notices also include the arrangements for services a resident will be receiving post transfer or discharge.

Transfer and discharge include any movement from the certified section of the nursing facility to the noncertified section of the facility and movement from the noncertified section of the facility to the certified section. Transfer and discharge include transfer to the hospital as well as community discharge.

If a resident appeals a decision, the facility cannot move the resident until the appeal is resolved through a fair hearing process. Residents have 30 days to make an appeal after receiving a transfer/discharge notice, or 14 days after an emergency discharge. The hearing decision is provided within a 45-day window. When a resident requests an expedited appeal, the hearing is scheduled as soon as possible (within a 7-day time frame), and a decision is made as soon as possible (within a 7-day time frame). Residents, in the expedited appeal, are notified verbally, approximately 48 hours before the hearing.

Use of Forms: All transfers/discharges in the nursing facility. These forms *are not* used for room changes on the same certified section of the facility.

Chart Location: These forms may be kept in a number of places. In the chart, the Misc. section or the Social Service section generally contain copies of these notices. Some facilities have separate binders to include copies of these notices. Other facilities keep the copies in the Social Service office resident file.

EXAMPLE OF 30-DAY NOTICE OF INTENT
TO TRANSFER/DISCHARGE RESIDENT

                                        (*Date of notice*)
Notice to: Copies to:
(*Name of resident*)   (*Name of representative*)

_____   _____

_____   _____

The purpose of this letter is to inform you that (*Name of nursing facility*) seeks to (*transfer/discharge*) you to (*Name of receiving facility, unit, or noninstitutional setting*) on (*date*). The reason(s) the nursing facility seeks to (*transfer/discharge*) you is/are:
(*Reason must be stated in specific detail*) _____

_____

The nursing facility has made arrangements for you to receive:
Services to be Provided: Name of Provider/Location of Discharge:

_____

YOU HAVE THE RIGHT TO APPEAL THE NURSING FACILITY'S PLAN TO TRANSFER OR DISCHARGE YOU. IF YOU DISAGREE WITH THIS DECISION, YOU MUST REQUEST A HEARING WITH THE DEPARTMENT OF PUBLIC WELFARE WITHIN 30 DAYS OF RECEIVING THIS NOTICE. IF YOU REQUEST A HEARING, YOU CANNOT BE TRANSFERRED OR DISCHARGED UNTIL 30 DAYS AFTER THE APPEAL DECISION IS RENDERED.

The person at the nursing facility who is responsible for supervising your transfer or discharge is _____. You should notify this person if you request an appeal or if you have any questions regarding this notice. You can send a request for a hearing by mail or fax. A hearing request form is enclosed with this notice. The nursing facility staff must help you in completing the request for a hearing if you request assistance.

You have the right to be represented at a hearing by an attorney or other advocate. For additional information or assistance, contact the following offices:

1. Local Long-Term Care Ombudsman Program
   (Address and telephone number)
2. Disability Law Center or Center for Public Representation (as appropriate)
   (Address and telephone number)
3. For free legal advice or representation, contact:
   Local Legal Services Office
   (Address and telephone number)

(Notice 1—Page 1)

EXAMPLE OF NOTICE OF NURSING FACILITY RESIDENT'S RIGHTS REGARDING A TRANSFER/DISCHARGE

You may only be transferred or discharged for one of the following reasons:

1) the move is necessary for your own welfare and your needs cannot be met within the nursing facility;
2) your health has improved sufficiently that you no longer need the services provided by the nursing facility;
3) the safety of individuals in the facility is endangered;
4) the health of individuals in the facility would otherwise be endangered;
5) you have failed, after reasonable and appropriate notice, to pay for (or failed to have Medicaid pay for) a stay in the facility; or
6) the facility is to be closed.

In general, you cannot be transferred or discharged until 30 days after you receive the nursing facility's notice, unless you agree to an earlier date. If you have resided in the nursing facility for less than 30 days, or your health has improved and you no longer need nursing care, or the health and safety of you or others in the facility is endangered, or you have urgent medical needs, the nursing facility can give you less than 30 days notice of its intent to transfer you and you will have the right to have an expedited appeal.

You have the right to appeal a nursing facility's plan to transfer or discharge you. You can file a request for a hearing with the department of Public Welfare's Division of Hearings. If you request an appeal prior to being moved, you cannot be transferred or discharged until after the hearing officer issues a decision in favor of the nursing facility. If the grounds for the planned transfer or discharge is nonpayment, you have the right to pay any amount owed. If you do this, the nursing facility may not transfer or discharge you for nonpayment.

If the hearing officer agrees with you, the nursing facility will not be permitted to transfer or discharge you. If the hearing officer decides in favor of the nursing facility, you will generally be allowed 30 days from the date you receive the decision to prepare for the move. If the reason for the transfer or discharge is one in which the nursing facility is allowed to give you less than 30 days notice, you will be allowed 5 days from the date you receive the decision to prepare for the move.

(Form 2—Page 1)

EXAMPLE OF A REQUEST FOR A HEARING

To be completed by the resident or the resident's representative:

(*Name and address of resident*)   (*Name and address of resident's representative*)

_____   _____

_____   _____

_____

(*Social Security Number of Resident*)

I WISH TO APPEAL THE PLAN OF (*Name of nursing facility*) TO TRANSFER OR DISCHARGE ME.

Attached is a copy of the transfer/discharge notice provided to me by the facility and received on (*Date*).

_____   _____

Date   Signature of Resident or Representative

Mail or fax this form to

DEPARTMENT OF PUBLIC WELFARE
DIVISION OF HEARINGS
P.O. BOX 167
ESSEX STATION
BOSTON, MA 02112-0167
FAX # (617) 727-9602

Give a copy of this form to the nursing facility contact person.

You will be notified by mail of the date, time, and hearing officer who will hear your appeal. Failure to appear at the hearing without good cause may result in dismissal of the appeal.

(Form 1—Page 1)

EXAMPLE OF NOTICE OF INTENT TO TRANSFER OR DISCHARGE RESIDENT WITH EXPEDITED APPEAL

(*Date of notice*)
Notice to: Copies to:
(*Name of resident*)   (*Name of representative*)

_____   _____

_____   _____

The purpose of this letter is to inform you that (*Name of nursing facility*) seeks to (*transfer/discharge*) you to (*Name of receiving facility, unit, or noninstitutional setting*) on (*Date*). The reason(s) the nursing facility seeks to (*transfer/discharge*) you is/are:
(*Reason must be stated in specific detail*) _____

_____

The nursing facility has made arrangements for you to receive:
Services to be Provided: Name of Provider/Location of Discharge:

_____

YOU HAVE THE RIGHT TO APPEAL THE NURSING FACILITY'S PLAN TO TRANSFER OR DISCHARGE YOU. IF YOU DISAGREE WITH THIS DECISION, YOU MUST REQUEST A HEARING WITH THE DEPARTMENT OF PUBLIC WELFARE WITHIN 14 DAYS OF RECEIVING THIS NOTICE. IF YOU REQUEST A HEARING, BEFORE BEING MOVED, YOU CANNOT BE MOVED UNTIL 5 DAYS AFTER YOU RECEIVE THE DECISION OF THE HEARING OFFICER.

If you have resided in the nursing facility for less than 30 days, or your health has improved and you no longer need nursing care, or the health and safety of you or others in the facility is endangered, or you have urgent medical needs, the nursing facility can give you less than a 30-day notice. In all other situations, the nursing facility must give you 30 days advance notice of its intent to transfer or discharge you.

The person at the nursing facility who is responsible for supervising your transfer or discharge is _____. You should notify this person if you request an appeal or if you have any questions regarding this notice. You can send a request for a hearing by mail or fax. A hearing request form is enclosed with this notice. The nursing facility staff must help you in completing the request for a hearing if you request assistance.

You have the right to be represented at a hearing by an attorney or other advocate. For additional information or assistance, contact the following offices:

1. Local Long Term Care Ombudsman Program
   (Address and telephone number)
2. Disability Law Center or Center for Public Representation (as appropriate)
   (Address and telephone number)
3. For free legal advice or representation contact:
   Local Legal Services Office
   (Address and telephone number

(Notice 2—Page 1)

Bed Hold Form

T he bed hold form[1] is used to inform residents and their designated
family members of their rights to hold a bed when there is a medical
leave of absence.

Copies to:

1. Resident
2. Family or responsible party
3. the chart

Use: Bed hold forms are required to be given at the time of transfer and
discharge. Notification of this process should be noted in the social service
notes in the chart.

Chart Location: The copies of these notices are often held in the Social Service
section, or in the Misc. section. Some facilities have copies in resident files in
the social service office.

---

[1]Some facilities have designed these forms to require signatures of receipt by residents or
family members.

BED HOLD POLICY AND NOTICE
(MASSACHUSETTS SAMPLE)

Date: _____
Resident name: _____
Transferred to: _____
Responsible party: _____
Address: _____

_____ 1. Medicaid: Residents covered by the Medicaid Program are entitled to a bed hold when they are transferred to a hospital or for a therapeutic leave of absence. Under the Medicaid Program, the duration of this bed hold for a medical leave of absence is up to 20 days. During this period, the resident is permitted to return and resume residence in the facility. For Medicaid recipients, private payment may be provided after 20 days for each day the bed is reserved. In the event that a bed is not reserved beyond a 20-day medical leave of absence, the resident is discharged. If the resident's hospitalization exceeds the bed hold period, the resident will be readmitted to (the nursing facility) of (town) immediately upon the first availability of an appropriate bed. This readmission is provided that the resident's needs may continue to be met by (nursing facility) and the resident is eligible for Medicaid services.

According to Massachusetts state Medicaid regulations, the duration of the bed hold is 20 days. Your bed hold period is from:
(A) Date of Transfer: _____
(B) Date of discharge: _____

_____ 2. Medicare or Private Insurance: Medicare and Private Insurances do not pay for a bed hold. Therefore, your bed hold will be based on your alternative funding source. Please see Medicaid Policy (#1) or Private Policy (#3).

_____ 3. Private Pay: For residents paying privately, payment must continue for all the days the bed is reserved. Unless otherwise notified, the facility will presume the bed is to be reserved, and the resident will pay for the full private rate during a medical leave of absence. The resident and/or responsible party may opt to cease a bed hold reservation at any time, in which case the resident will be discharged and the room vacated of personal belongs (which will be stored according to nursing facility policies).

According to the Private Plan, your bed hold period begins on:
Date of Transfer: _____

I agree to pay the private or the semi-private room rate of $_____ per day for name of resident, while he/she is hospitalized. I was notified by telephone on _____.

Signature: _____
Date: _____
Relationship to resident: _____

Community Discharge Plan Form

T his is a form devised to assist social workers in their discharge of residents to the community.

The uses of this form are as

- a discharge planning worksheet;
- a comprehensive planning tool with residents and families;
- a planning tool with other staff members.

Chart location: Generally this form would be in the social service office file or in the Social Service section of the resident chart.

COMMUNITY DISCHARGE PLAN

Name: _____

Address: _____   Phone: _____

❐ Notice of discharge (expedited) given with resident rights and 30-day readmittance

Date: _____

The following areas may be included in the resident discharge plan:

1. Facility physician's order for discharge: _____

   ❐ Name of attending physician in the community: _____

   Phone # _____

   3 Page Referral(s)

   ❐ Fax 3-page referral   ❐ Resident hand carry home referral
   ❐ Mailed referral

2. Medications:

   ❐ Medications given at time of discharge   # of days: _____
   (See nursing page 1)

3. Financial arrangements for all community services:

   ❐ Medicare to pay for continuing care needs
   ❐ Medicaid
   ❐ Private insurance   ❐ Private pay

4. Transportation to home:

   ❐ family/friend car   ❐ ambulance   ❐ other: _____
   ❐ wheelchair van   ❐ taxi

5. Home care services:

   ❐ Visiting Nurses   ❐ Elder Services

   Date service to begin: _____   Date service to begin: _____

   ❐ Physical Therapy   ❐ Meals on Wheels
   ❐ Occupational Therapy   ❐ Homemaker
   ❐ Home Health Aide   ❐ Other: _____
   ❐ Social Worker: _____
   ❐ Hospice   ❐ Assisted Living Setting

6. Special equipment at time of discharge:

   ❐ Walker   ❐ Bathtub bench   Where
                                         delivered: _____
   ❐ Cane   ❐ Grab bars   Date to be
                                         delivered: _____
   ❐ Wheelchair   ❐ Oxygen
   ❐ Commode   ❐ Other: _____

7. Emergency Home Medical system:

❐ Type: _____   ❐ Date service to start: _____

8. Family available to assist with:
   ❐ Meet at facility and assist with discharge
   ❐ Meal preparation   ❐ Medication monitoring
   ❐ Transportation   ❐ Finances
   ❐ Other: _____

Key family members:

EMB 10/2001

Interdisciplinary Team Meeting Record

This form is an outline for the interdisciplinary team to follow during their meetings together. It helps to identify and focus the meeting function, and provides a record of the meeting for the chart.

Use: Quarterly and interim meetings of the interdisciplinary team.

Chart Location: This form would be in the care plan section of the chart. If the care plans are stored in a separate binder, this form would be located with the current care plans.

INTERDISCIPLINARY TEAM MEETING RECORD

Resident Name: _____   Date: ___ / ___ / ___

    Admission MDS: ☐   Quarterly Review: ☐   Annual MDS: ☐
    Significant Change: ☐   Significant Correction: ☐   Other: ☐

Brief Summary of Meeting:

_____

_____

Physical Restraint Reviewed/Discussed:	Yes ☐ No ☐	N/A ☐	Current Consent ☐
Chemical Restraint Reviewed/Discussed:	Yes ☐ No ☐	N/A ☐	Current Consent ☐
Self-Medication Reviewed/ Discussed:	Yes ☐ No ☐	N/A ☐	Current Consent ☐
Advance Directives Status Discussed:	Yes ☐ No ☐		Current Consent ☐
DNR Status (including community) Discussed:	Yes ☐ No ☐		Current Consent ☐
Face Sheet Checked for Accuracy	Yes ☐ No ☐		
Current LTC Screening Form in Chart	Yes ☐ No ☐	N/A ☐	
Current Guardianships, Including Roger's, in Chart	Yes ☐ No ☐	N/A ☐	
Current Health Care Proxy in Chart	Yes ☐ No ☐		
Medical Record Purged per Policy, for Outdated, Nonvalid Consents:	Yes ☐ No ☐		

Attendance:

Name	*Title*	*Discipline*

Estimated Length of Stay: _____
Submitted by: _____   Title: _____

Nursing Home Social Work Practice Standards: An Example From Massachusetts[1]

INTRODUCTION

In 1991, the NASW Nursing Home Committee of Massachusetts made a decision by which they hoped to impact the practice of social work in nursing homes throughout the Commonwealth of Massachusetts. The Committee decided to develop its own Practice Standards rather than rely on the State or the nursing home industry. This development was preceded by over 12 years of work by the Committee with the Department of Public Health in an attempt to formulate new State regulations regarding social work practice in nursing homes.

The work was abandoned by the State following the election of a new governor. This disappointment led the committee to empower the social work community to take charge of their own professional destiny and to develop their own standards. The Committee began its work by forming a Practice Standards Sub-Committee, composed of social workers from different geographical areas. One of the primary goals was to involve as a many social workers as possible, so they could claim ownership in the project. This was accomplished through the participation of hundreds of social workers for a 4-year period. Regional social workers from the Berkshires to Cape Cod drafted different sections of the document, which were reviewed by the Sub-Committee.

There was an ongoing exchange of material between the groups. This work was supplemented by the involvement of participants at the Annual Nursing Home Social Work Conference, which is attended by over 300 people. Attendees provided the Sub-Committee with comments, which were reviewed and evaluated. The project culminated with a series of seven statewide hearings, which were attended by over 140 social workers. The material from the hearings was evaluated and incorporated into a final draft. This was adopted by the Executive Committee and the Board of Directors of The Massachusetts Chapter of NASW.

---

[1]Reprinted with permission from NASW Massachusetts Chapter, © 1997.

These Standards provide the reader with a foundation for social work practice in the nursing home. They are not intended to be a manual about how to practice social work in the nursing home. How social workers practice is dependent upon individual experiences, education, and levels of competency. These standards begin with a preamble, which is an overview of the document. It is followed by five basic social work functions. They are administration, advocacy, clinical, consultation, and education. It concludes with personnel practices. Each section has an introduction that provides the rationale for the standard and is followed by an interpretation.

In conclusion, these Practice Standards are a constant in the midst of an ever-changing health care system. The industry has seen the birth of Medicare, Medicaid, and Managed Health Care. The challenges faced by social workers, health care professionals, and consumers is to maintain these standards which strive to assure humane and compassionate treatment of nursing home residents and their families.

—The Practice Standards Committee
Ed Alessi
Frank Baskin, Project Coordinator
Diane Finnemore
Carolyn Sones

PRACTICE STANDARDS

PREAMBLE

The nursing home social worker is mandated to adhere to the professional code of Ethics of the National Association of Social Workers. We have a legal obligation to adhere to governmental laws. We have a professional responsibility to provide good service, and to bring about change when laws unjustly affect our client population. We are responsible for fostering a climate, policies, and routines, which enable residents to retain individuality, independence, and dignity.

ADMINISTRATION

Introduction

The Social Worker shall carry out administrative functions in order to meet the needs of residents.

Standard A

The social worker shall participate in the development and implementation of policies regarding resident care, social work practice, and personnel policies.

Interpretation

1. The Social Worker shall be a part of the interdisciplinary team that meets regularly to review facilities' policies and procedures regarding compliance with State and Federal Regulations.
2. The Social Worker shall influence policies that affect resident care and the quality of residents' lives.
3. The Social Worker shall be involved with the development of policies that affect social service job descriptions, employment criteria, work standards, job benefits.

Standard B

The Social Worker shall be knowledgeable of and maintain regular contact with all community resources.

Interpretation

1. The Social Worker shall develop a knowledge base of community resources which are available to the long-term care residents as well as those residents with discharge potential.
2. The Social Worker shall assume a proactive role in the supporting and utilizing of community resources.
3. The Social Worker shall maintain a current resource file.
4. The Social Worker shall educate the community regarding the nursing home as a resource.

Standard C

The Social Worker shall participate in quality assurance in order to assure effective practice of social work in meeting residents' needs.

Interpretation

1. The Social Worker shall participate in regular quality assurance interdisciplinary team meetings.
2. The Social Worker shall identify problems and develop and implement studies relative to issues affecting residents.
3. The Social Worker shall develop recommendations resulting from quality assurance data.

Standard D

The Social Worker shall understand and meet all government requirements for social service documentation.

ADVOCACY

Introduction

The Social Worker shall be an advocate who promotes self-advocacy for residents and an increased awareness of issues that impact on the quality of life of nursing home residents.

Standard A

The Social Worker shall be knowledgeable of nursing home, community, and governmental practices that directly or indirectly affect nursing home residents.

Interpretation

1. The Social Worker shall work with the interdisciplinary team and administration to promote and protect residents' rights and the psychosocial well-being of each resident.
2. The Social worker has legal and professional responsibility to prevent and address resident abuse.
3. The Social Worker shall identify community changes and opportunities such as legislation, regulations, and programs that affect nursing homes residents.

Standard B

The Social Worker shall assist residents, family/significant others, and staff on how to effectively advocate for the residents.

Interpretation

The Social Worker shall work with residents, family/significant others, and staff individually or in groups to provide support, information, and organization for taking a more proactive role in making changes which improve the quality of life for individual residents as well as within the nursing home and in the community.

CLINICAL

Introduction

The Social Worker shall be responsible for doing psychosocial assessment, social history, care planning, and clinical interventions with residents and family/significant others in order to alleviate social and emotional problems.

Standard A

The Social Worker shall develop individualized, comprehensive psychosocial assessments for each resident.

Interpretation

1. The Social Worker shall record and develop psychosocial history and assessments in a timely fashion to be a part of the resident's permanent record.
2. The Social Worker shall include the resident, family members, significant others, and referral sources as sources of data.
3. The Social Worker shall consider the following: identifying data, cultural and background information, personal characteristics, interpersonal relationships, functioning levels, orientation, attitudes, decision-making abilities, mental status, coping, behavior patterns, and legal issues.
4. The Social Worker shall develop discharge planning to reflect the resident's potential to return to the community.
5. The Social Worker shall assess the needs and nature of counseling for residents including the use of community mental health services.

Standard B

The Social Worker shall participate in the development of an interdisciplinary treatment plan for each resident.

Interpretation

1. The plan shall include: identified psychosocial problems of resident, family and significant others insofar as they impact on the resident; short- and long-term goals which attempt to resolve identified problems; approaches for social work intervention.
2. Discharge planning and referrals to community resources (as appropriate).
3. Residents and their family/significant others shall be encouraged to participate in the formulation process, ongoing evaluation, and reassessment with the interdisciplinary team.

Standard C

The Social Worker shall ensure the appropriate provision of counseling services for residents with identified psychosocial needs.

Interpretation

1. Individual, group, and family treatment modalities shall be utilized.
2. During the initial period following admission the Social Worker shall provide intensive and frequent contacts with the resident and family/ significant others.
3. The Social Worker shall provide time-limited counseling services to residents as deemed appropriate.
4. The Social Worker shall refer to appropriate community mental health services.

CONSULTATION

Introduction

Social service consultation shall be provided on a planned basis with sufficient frequency to enable the Social Worker, administration, and facility staff to meet the psychosocial needs of residents.

Standard A

The consultant shall provide clinical consultation to the staff Social Worker.

Interpretation

1. The Social Worker shall review clinical services focusing on psychodynamics, delivery, and documentation of services.
2. The consultant shall assist the staff Social Worker to further develop and maximize skills in interviewing, assessment, recording, and treatment modalities.

Standard B

The consultant shall provide general consultation to the staff Social Worker.

Interpretation

1. The consultant shall discuss administrative and organizational issues; program planning, professional development and long-term care issues.
2. The consultant shall provide support to the Social Worker and enable the Social Worker to self-advocate.

Standard C

The consultant shall provide consultation to the administration.

Interpretation

1. The consultant shall discuss program planning, policy development, and priority setting regarding social services.
2. The consultant shall review the function and role of the staff Social Worker (including personnel issues).
3. The consultant shall advocate for social services with administration and other staff members.

Standard D

The consultant shall provide consultation to the facility staff.

Interpretation

1. The consultant shall be available to provide case consultation regarding psychosocial needs of resident and family/significant others.
2. The consultant shall provide in-service education to the staff on selected topics or clinical concerns.

EDUCATION

Introduction

The Social Worker shall educate resident, family/significant others, and staff in order to create an atmosphere where residents are cared for, respected, and appreciated as individuals.

Standard A

The Social Worker shall educate nursing home staff on an ongoing basis regarding the Social Worker's role in the facility and the psychosocial needs of residents and their family/significant others.

Interpretation

The Social Worker shall have regular contact with nursing home staff and participate in periodic planned in-services. This allows the Social Worker to help sensitize the staff to

1. The psychosocial problems of aging, illness, and disability, both in general and how they specifically impact a particular resident or family member.
2. The importance of each staff member's involvement in caring for residents.
3. An awareness of cultural diversity.
4. The role of the Social Worker.

Standard B

The Social Worker shall educate residents and family/significant others about living in a nursing home setting and the options available to them.

Interpretation

The Social Worker shall have regular contact with residents and their family/ significant others to help them understand

1. Their rights and responsibilities.
2. How to problem-solve when conflicts arise.
3. What community, social, and health services are available to them, including discharge planning.

Standard C

The Social Worker shall supervise students assigned to social services.

Interpretation

1. The Social Worker shall assign tasks in accordance with guidelines from the student's school.
2. The Social Worker shall be accountable for the student's work and documentation.

PERSONNEL PRACTICES

Introduction

The Social Worker shall be in compliance with government regulations and shall adhere to the professional code of ethics of NASW and the Social Work Licensing Boards. The Social Worker shall be provided with the necessary administrative support in order to carry out the Social Work mission.

Standard A

Any Social Worker who staffs a long-term care facility shall have a license in the Commonwealth of Massachusetts at the Licensed Social Worker (LSW) or higher level of licensure.

Interpretation

1. The Social Worker shall be licensed in accordance with state and federal regulations.
2. The minimum number of Social Worker hours per week shall be determined on a ratio of 1 social work hour per 1.5 residents.
3. Frequent transfers, admissions, and discharges shall warrant an increase in social work hours per resident.

Standard B

The Social Worker shall receive supervision by a licensed MSW Social Worker (LICSW or LICSW eligible).

Interpretation

The number of hours per month of supervision shall be based on a minimum ration of 1 hour of supervision to every 5 hours of social work per week.

Standard C

The Social Worker shall meet the requirement for continuing education as designated by the Commonwealth.

Interpretation

1. The Social Worker shall be provided with the opportunity to complete continuing education requirements in order to maintain his/her social work license.
2. The Social Worker shall be reimbursed by the employer and be provided the time to attend educational programs that shall benefit the facility and enhance his/her practice.

Standard D

The Social Worker shall engage in activities which shall increase professional knowledge and enhance professional development.

Interpretation

1. The Social worker shall expand knowledge and skills levels to increase the level of proficiency in carrying out the identified social work roles.
2. The Social Worker shall have access to adequate and updated written material pertinent to the performance and enhancement of the social work function.
3. The Social Worker shall be provided with the time and opportunity to participate in professional organizations and to network with colleagues.

Standard E

The Social Worker shall require adequate supplies, clerical services, and office space to effectively and adequately carry out the social work functions.

Interpretation

1. The Social Worker shall have a quiet, comfortable, secure, private, furnished, and handicapped accessible office. This shall ensure confidentiality for residents, family, and staff.
2. The Social Worker shall have a secure file cabinet in the office to maintain confidentiality of records.
3. The Social Worker shall have a telephone and have access to other modes of communication (fax machine, computers, etc.) in order to effectively carry out his/her responsibilities.
4. The Social Worker shall be provided with adequate clerical services.

Standard F

The nursing home shall have written policies in place which describe the contact between the Social Worker and the nursing home in order to identify mutual expectations during the Social Worker's employment.

Interpretation

1. A written contract shall identify the terms of employment between the Social Worker and the nursing home.
2. The Social Worker's immediate supervisor shall provide an annual written and oral evaluation of the Social Worker.

Quarterly Social Service Note Form

This form can be used to write quarterly progress notes or as reminder of areas to address within written progress notes. Interim notes should be written aside and provide backup to quarterly notes.

Use: 90-day review of resident progress toward goal(s).

Chart location: Quarterly notes are in the social service section of the chart. Generally, they are kept in chronological order, the last note at the back of the section. Quarterly notes of 2 to 3 years duration are generally kept.

SOCIAL SERVICE QUARTERLY PROGRESS NOTE

Date of Review: _____

Resident Name: _____   Room #: _____

Date of Birth: _____   Last Admission Date: _____

Hospitalizations during past quarter:

Mental Illness Diagnosis:	Yes ☐	No ☐
Developmental Disability Diagnosis:	Yes ☐	No ☐
Psych. Services:	Yes ☐	No ☐
Last Date of Service: _____		
Counseling:	Yes ☐	No ☐
Medication Review:	Yes ☐	No ☐
Family Meetings During Last Quarter:	Yes ☐	No ☐
Room Changes:	Yes ☐	No ☐
Roommate Changes:	Yes ☐	No ☐
Pain Management:	Yes ☐	No ☐
Hospice:	Yes ☐	No ☐

Current Resident Status, Including Mental State, Physical Condition, Improvements or Deterioration:

Resident Discharge Potential:

Progress Toward Social Service Identified Goal(s):

New Goals: Yes ☐   No ☐

_____

Social Service Signature and Title

EMB 5/99

Social Service Evaluation Form

This is a sample form which can be utilized to evaluate the performance of a social worker within the Social Service Department. The focus is on social work skills within the role.

Use: This form can be utilized by the facility Administrator or the Director of Social Services as a part of the annual or biannual performance review of the facility social worker.

Place Located: The evaluation can be held in the personnel file of the social worker, as well as the worker having her own copy.

Caution: This should be a confidential evaluation, to be shared with only the Director of Social Services, the Administrator and the social worker who is being evaluated.

SOCIAL SERVICE EVALUATION

Facility: _____
Name: _____   Date of Evaluation: _____
Position: _____   Date of Hire: _____

Range of Evaluation: *Excellent, Good, Fair, Poor*

1. **Ability to establish and maintain meaningful, effective, appropriately professional relationships with client system.**
   A. Attitudes as manifested in appropriate behavior toward client:
      Interest and desire to be helpful   _____
      Empathic understanding   _____
      Nonjudgmental acceptance   _____
      Assent to client self-determination   _____
      Warmth and concern   _____
      Respect   _____
   B. Objective, disciplined use of self in relationship on
      behalf of clients: Empathy and sympathy without over-iden-   _____
      tification
   C. Adherence to professionally accepted value in client
      contact: Confidentiality   _____

2. **Social work process—knowledge and skills.**
   A. Information gathering skills:
      Ability to gather relevant information from client   _____
      Observation and exploration of relevant items are accurate   _____
      and appropriately detailed
      Discrimination ability to discern psychosocial factors of   _____
      significance that need to be explored
   B. Assessment skills:
      Effectively applied knowledge of human behavior and so-   _____
      cial systems so as to derive meanings from information
      gathering
      Shows appreciation and understanding of client's percep-   _____
      tual cognitive and emotional frame of reference
      Capable of formulating a descriptive, dynamic information   _____
      assessment statement
   C. Intervention skills:
      To plan and implement a program of remediation based   _____
      on assessment
      Ability to use specific treatment interventions, as appro-   _____
      priate to client's situation
      Interventions are appropriately timed and relevant   _____
   D. Interviewing skills:
      Ability to establish with client clear interview purpose   _____
      Ability to maintain interview focus in order to attain inter-   _____
      view purpose
      Maintains a good balance; flexibility; responsibly following   _____

client lead and offering appropriate directions and control

Ability to tactfully and nonthreateningly help client communicate feelings as well as facts   _____

   E. Recording skills:

Timely   _____

Coordinates with other team members   _____

Content   _____

3. Facility.

Knowledge of, commitment to, and identification with facility objectives, policies, and procedures   _____

Ability to work within the limits of facility policies and procedures   _____

4. Supervision.

   A. Administrative aspects:

Prepares adequately for conference, provides supervisor with necessary, appropriate material for conference   _____

   B. Interpersonal aspects:

Seeks and uses supervisor's help without undue dependency   _____

Acceptance of supervision and instruction, positive orientation to supervisory authority   _____

Ability to recognize when consultation is needed and how it might be appropriately used   _____

5. Staff and community relationships.

Contributes to harmonious and effective relationships with facility staff at all levels   _____

Develops positive relationships with and makes appropriate use of colleagues from allied disciplines   _____

Constructively represents the facility to other professionals and to the general public   _____

Has good knowledge of relevant community resources   _____

6. Management of work requirements and work load.

Covers work load with regularity and adequacy   _____

Shows ability to plan and organize work schedule within time allotted   _____

Shows capacity to set selective, valid priorities, and to schedule work accordingly   _____

Is prompt in submitting reports and recording   _____

7. Professionally related attributes and attitudes.

Realistic critical assessment of own limitations without undue anxiety   _____

Adequate level of self-awareness and capacity for self-evaluation   _____

Flexible and cooperative on the job   _____

Behaves on the job in accordance with the values and ethics _____
of the profession
Provides creative solutions to problems _____

Comments:

Evaluation submitted by: _____
Reviewed with Social Worker: _____

Social Service Job Description Sample

Social Service Department
Job: Director of Social Services
Reporting to: Facility Administrator

Statement of Purpose:

The social worker in _____ is to provide social services to residents in the nursing facility through the identification of the resident's psychosocial, mental, and emotional needs and provide or aid in the access of services to meet these needs. The focus is to provide the highest practical level of physical, mental, and psychosocial well-being, and quality of life attainable by the facility residents.

Qualifications:

The incumbent must be a social worker who holds the minimum of a Bachelor's degree in Social Work, Psychology, Human Services, or other related field and who is licensed (or license eligible) in Massachusetts at the Licensed Social Worker (LSW) level. MSW Consultation, as per Massachusetts Department of Public Health regulations, provided for social workers holding a bachelor's degree. The social worker should have a minimum of 2–3 years of experience working with elders, preferably in long-term care, and competent social work skills.

Additional Qualifications:

Incumbents must have skills in communication, assessment, and social work methods and techniques. Incumbents should have the skills to provide support groups to resident, families, or staff as needed. As of December 25, 1998, incumbents must also pass a "CORI" check in Massachusetts.

Primary Duties:

The social work department is responsible for a psychosocial assessment evaluation and development plan of care for all newly admitted residents that may include but is not limited to:

- addressing resident's emotional and social factors relating to medical condition or treatment;
- resident's personal or interpersonal problems, issues, or needs while in the nursing facility;
- identifying present or future adjustment difficulties;
- addressing the probable length of stay;
- implementing varied approaches with staff to meet resident's needs;
- casework and group work as identified to resolve any social or emotional problems;
- community referrals as directed by resident need;
- assisting to obtain for the resident financial, legal, or community services as needed;
- acting as a liaison between the resident and the mental health agency/provider;
- attending URC, Ethics Committee, Interdisciplinary, Administrative staff meetings and other meetings as requested;
- participating in, developing programs for Quality Assurance in the facility;
- checking departmental documentation periodically to ensure all records are in compliance with Federal/State regulations;
- developing department policies and procedures of the Social Service Department and reviewing these annually making necessary changes and upgrades as needed;
- coordinating staff and family groups as needed.

Documentation:

The social work department provides timely entries in the resident's chart to include, but not limited to: a social service history of each resident as well as a psychosocial assessment. A care plan is formulated for each resident addressing problems, needs, and interventions. Documentation is provided to substantiate interventions, progress toward, and/or completion of goals. Documentation includes information pertaining to residents who are transferred from the facility.

Department Reporting:

The Social Service Department prepares and provides monthly reports of activities for the Facility Administrator.

Discharge Planning:

Each resident will be assessed by the Social Service Department, as a member of the interdisciplinary team, for discharge. The Social Service Department will assist with plans for the resident's discharge and post-discharge with the resident, family, interdisciplinary team, and community resources. He or she will assist the resident and/or family in the implementation of the discharge plan and orientation around this process.

In-Service Training and Education:

In-service training is provided, on a continuing basis, for all the staff at the facility. This training, conducted by the social worker, deals with the orientation of the facility staff toward the creation of therapeutic community, congenial atmosphere, and healthy interpersonal relationships; enhances staff understanding of the normal aging process as well as issues around illness, need for dignity, quality of life, and placement. Training also instills the need, and the insight into, early recognition and treatment of psychosocial problems. Training and education will be offered to the community at large around issues of aging, rights of residents, facility services, and other related topics.

The social worker will continue to pursue education to increase own knowledge and skills.

Resident's Rights:

In-services are provided regularly by the Social Service Department for all staff on Resident's Rights and Abuse, Neglect, and Mistreatment, mandatory reporting law, as well as the facility policies regarding implementing these issues. The social worker acts as the resident's advocate.

Health Care Proxy Form (Massachusetts and New York)

The Health Care Proxy form allows a resident (principal) to select a person to have the authority to make health care decisions for them. The Health Care Proxy is not effective until the resident (principal) is determined, by their attending physician, in writing, to no longer have the capacity to make those decisions.

Uses: This form is used when the resident is determined to be no longer capable of making health care decisions for themself including such issues as life-sustaining treatment or psychoactive medication. The Health Care Proxy is the recognized instrument for making Advance Directives.

Chart Location: The Health Care Proxy is generally found in the Legal section of the chart. Some charts have plastic sleeves that protect this type of document. Occasionally, this type of document will be kept with the admission paperwork.

MASSACHUSETTS HEALTH CARE PROXY

1. I, _____,

(Principal—PRINT your name)

residing at _____

(Street)   (City or Town)   (State)

appoint as my Health Care Agent: _____

(Name of person you choose as Agent)

of _____

(Street)   (City or Town)   (State)   (Phone number)

(Optional; If my agent is unwilling or unable to serve, then I appoint as my Alternate:

_____, of

_____.)

(Street)   (City or Town)   (State)   (Phone number)

2. My Agent shall have the authority to make all health care decisions for me, including decisions about life-sustaining treatment, subject to any limitations I state below, if I am unable to make health care decisions myself. My Agent's authority becomes effective if my attending physician determines in writing that I lack the capacity to make or to communicate health care decisions. My Agent is then to have the same authority to make health care decisions as I would if I had the capacity to make them except (here list the limitations if any, you wish to place on your Agent's authority):

I direct my Agent to make health care decisions based on my Agent's assessment of my personal wishes. If my personal wishes are unknown, my Agent is to make health care decisions based on my Agent's assessment of my best interests. Photocopies of this Health Care Proxy shall have the same force and effect as the original.

3. Signed: _____

Complete only if Principal is physically unable to sign: I have signed the Principal's name above at his/her direction in the presence of the Principal and two witnesses.

_____   _____

Name   Street

_____

City or Town   State

4. WITNESS STATEMENT: We, the undersigned, each witnessed the signing of this Health Care Proxy by the Principal or at the direction of the Principal and state that the Principal appears to be at least 18 years of age, of sound mind and under no constraints or undue influence. Neither of us is named as the Health Care Agent or Alternative in this document.

In our presence this _____ day of _____, _____.

Witness #1 _____   Witness #2 _____
    Signature   Signature

Name: _____   Name: _____
    Print   Print

Address: _____   Address: _____

_____   _____

5. Statements of Health Care Agent and Alternate (Optional):
Health Agent: I have been named by the Principal as the Principal's Health Care Agent by this Health Care Proxy. I have read this document carefully, and have personally discussed with the Principal his/her health care wishes at a time of possible incapacity. I know the Principal and accept this appointment freely. I am not an operator, administrator, or employee of a hospital, clinic, nursing home, rest home, Soldiers Home, or other health care facility where the Principal is presently a patient or resident or has applied for admission. Or if I am a person so described, I am also related to the Principal by blood, marriage or adoption. If I called upon and to the best of my ability, I will try to carry out the Principal's wishes.

Signature of Health Care Agent: _____

Alternate: I have been named by the Principal as the Principal's Alternate by this Health Care Proxy. I have read this document carefully, and have personally discussed with the Principal his/her health care wishes at a time of possible incapacity. I know the Principal and accept this appointment freely. I am not an operator, administrator, or employee of a hospital, clinic, nursing home, rest home, Soldiers Home, or other health care facility where the Principal is presently a patient or resident or has applied for admission. Or if I am a person so described, I am also related to the Principal by blood, marriage, or adoption. If I am called upon and to the best of my ability, I will try to carry out the Principal's wishes.

Signature of Alternate: _____

NEW YORK STATE HEALTH CARE PROXY

(1) I, _____, hereby appoint
(name) _____
(address) _____
(telephone number) _____
as my health care agent to make any and all health care decisions for me, except to the extent that I state otherwise. This proxy shall take effect when and if I become unable to make my own health care decisions.

(2) Optional instructions: I direct my agent to make health care decisions in accord with my wishes and limitations as stated below, or as he or she otherwise knows. (Attach additional pages if necessary.)

_____
_____
_____

(Unless your agent knows your wishes about artificial nutrition and hydration [feeding tubes], your agent will not be allowed to make decisions about artificial nutrition and hydration. See instructions on reverse for samples of language you could use.)

(3) Name of substitute or fill-in agent if the person I appoint above is unable, unwilling, or unavailable to act as my health care agent:
(name) _____
(address) _____
(telephone number) _____

(4) Unless I revoke it, this proxy shall remain in effect indefinitely, or until the date or conditions stated below. This proxy shall expire (specific date or conditions, if desired):

_____

(5) Signature _____
Address _____
Date _____

Statement by Witnesses (must be 18 or older)

I declare that the person who signed this document is personally known to me and appears to be of sound mind and acting of his or her own free will. He or she signed (or asked another to sign for him or her) this document in my presence.
Witness 1 _____
Witness 2 _____
Witness 3 _____
Address _____

Afterword: Advocacy, Research, and the Nursing Home Social Worker

A review of the literature demonstrates that a great deal has been written about the elderly, the long-term care field, and nursing facilities. Very little has been written or researched, however, about the capacity of social workers to effectively intervene to help meet the psychosocial needs of nursing home residents. It is important for nursing facility social workers to engage in this research and investigation to address the day-to-day problems and solutions of residents and their families. The social workers' direct knowledge of resident/family needs can be an essential ingredient for successful research.

As social workers in nursing facilities face the increasing complex health care issues of the new millennium, the need for outcomes-based research will also increase. Decisions for staffing and expenditures for services will be based upon the demonstrated results of research, projects, and grants. The emphasis is on the interdisciplinary team, of which social workers are an important component in meeting the needs of, and assuring a quality of life for residents.

Nursing home social workers can join with others in local or regional groups. Statewide or national committees can offer support or resources to long-term care facility social workers as well. These groups can encourage and support the role of the social worker in the nursing home facility through continuing education programs, ongoing research, and legislative lobbying. Sponsorship for activities can occur through such organizations as the National Association of Social Workers, Association for Gerontology Education in Social Work, Gerontological Society of America, Council on Social Work Education/SAGE-SW, National Alliance for Caregiving, National Council on the Aging, and Administration on Aging.

Advocacy of the social work role in the facility is essential. Elders and their family members benefit substantially from having professional social workers with expertise and skill assisting them through issues brought about through illness and the need for nursing care. I urge you to take an active role in advocating, promoting, and sustaining social work in nursing facilities. It is through the dedication of social workers that the lives of our residents are ultimately enriched and valued.

Glossary of Commonly Used Terms and Abbreviations

ADL	Activities of Daily Living
BID	Twice a day
BP	Blood pressure
c	with
Care Plans	Residents have an individual interdisciplinary plan of care for all their problems and needs. This includes identification of a specific problem or need; a succinct, measurable, time-specific goal; and intervention(s) by team members.
Case Mix Reimbursement	A system for reimbursing nursing home services that reflects the specific patient care needs of the residents.
Case Mix System	The database storing all Management Minutes Questionnaires data that will be used for administrative and quality monitoring purposes.
c/o	complaints of
D/C	discontinue
Dx	Diagnosis
FBS	fasting blood sugar
fx	fracture
HCFA	Health Care Financing Administration
hs	hour of sleep or bedtime
Hx	history
I & O	Intake and output
IM	intramuscular

inc	incontinent
JCAHO	Joint Commission Accreditation of Health Organizations
LTC	Long-Term Care
lg	large
Managed Minutes	A method of measuring case mix by assigning weights to discrete caregiving activities or to characteristics of patients found to require given amounts of care. The Managed Minutes Data System is the organized procedure for collecting, storing, and analyzing this information.
Medicaid	(Title XIX of the Social Security Act). The federal and state funded grant program, and state-administrated health care program to provide indigent people (both young and old) access to health care. Each state sets the individual income and asset guidelines in order for individuals to qualify for the program.
Medicare	(Title XVIII of the Social Security Act). Parts A & B—Premiums paid for by participants as this is both an entitlement and insurance program. Individuals qualify by having worked within the Social Security system, or being disabled and meeting qualifications.
MDS	Minimum Data Set (2.0). This form provides a core set of clinical and functional status screening elements that form the foundation of the comprehensive assessment.
nf	nursing facility
NGT	nasal gastric tube
noc	night
NPO	nothing by mouth
OBRA	Omnibus Reconciliation Act of 1987 that was implemented across the country in 1989, making enormous, sweeping changes and additions to the regulation of long-term care.
OSCAR	Standard Reports #3 and #4 from HCFA's Online Survey, Certification and Reporting system. Report #3 gives the state surveyor a history of the facility in profile per the last four previous surveys as well as additional complaints, problems, and corrections. Report #4 provides the surveyors with the facility's physical plant problems and corrections, if any.
OT	Occupational Therapy
PASARR	The OBRA acronym for Preadmission Screening and Annual Resident Review. The requirements of §483.100–§483.136 govern the State's responsibility for preadmission screening

and annual resident review of individuals with mental illness and mental retardation.

PNA   Personal Needs Account. This is money left in an account in the facility for the resident. Medicaid currently provides eligible residents in nursing facilities with a monthly amount determined by each individual state.

po   by mouth

PPS   Prospective Payment System for Medicare participating facilities. This means that the facilities, based upon preset rates and codes are paid by Medicare in a lump sum for care of eligible residents.

prn   as needed

pt   patient

PT   Physical Therapy

qd   every day

qh   every hour

qid   four times a day

qod   every other day

RAI   Resident Assessment Instrument. A standard, structured approach for applying a problem identification model in long-term care facilities.

RAP   Resident Assessment Protocol

RUGS-s III   Resource Utilization Groups. This is a patient classification system that identifies the relative costs (resource costs) of providing care for different types of patients based upon their resource use.

Rx   treatment

s   without

SNF   Skill Nursing Facility

SOB   shortness of breath

ST   speech therapy

TID   three times a day

TPR   temperature, pulse, respiration

vd   voided

w/c   wheelchair

Index

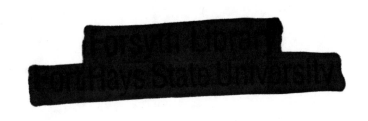
Forsyth Library
Fort Hays State University